Helen Keller

Other titles in *Heroes of the Cross* series

To be published shortly:

Helen Keller

Catherine M. Swift

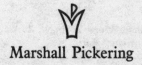

Marshall Pickering

Marshall Morgan and Scott
Marshall Pickering
34–42 Cleveland Street, London W1P 5FB, U.K.

ISBN: 0 551 02028-8

Text Set in Plantin by Avocet Robinson, Buckingham
Printed and bound in Great Britain by
Cox & Wyman Ltd, Reading

Contents

Introduction

Before reading the story of Helen Keller it is essential to try to understand precisely how her condition affected her. I say *try* because it is impossible for anyone not similarly afflicted to capture fully the extent of her childhood sufferings.

If we place our hands over our ears and close our eyes tightly we can still see images and hear sounds because our memories reproduce them. But as Helen lost her sight and hearing when a baby, she soon outgrew her memories and before very long had none to recall.

Also she was unable to speak because there was no way of teaching her words when she could neither see nor hear.

Whenever reference is made in this book to her mother, father or anyone else, this is for the reader's benefit because Helen never knew them as such. People, animals and things didn't have names. She didn't even know the words 'people', 'animals' or 'things'. How could she when no one had the means of telling or showing her anything?

In her black and silent world she was left with only smell, touch and taste so, although her doll was named Nancy, Helen didn't know that — or even that it was *a doll*. And with her mind completely empty of words she couldn't *think*, I'm hungry – cold – tired – happy – miserable or ill.

1

Heartbreak

Arthur Keller, a retired American Confederate Army Captain, was devoted to his family. Since his retirement from the army he had become editor of a local newspaper and though he had an office in the nearby town of Tuscumbia, he worked largely from home. A warm-hearted person with many friends, he liked nothing better than to entertain them at his lovely old farmhouse in North West Alabama, one of the southern most states of America.

Situated by the Tennessee River on the outskirts of Tuscumbia — meaning Great Spring to the Indians — Ivy Green was an enormous house with many spacious rooms and, in typical southern fashion, it was fronted by a wooden verandah. Festooned with honeysuckle and rambling roses, the verandah overlooked sweeping lawns surrounded by flowering trees and shrubs; violets, lilies, roses and almost every other blossom imaginable. And with ivy covering the walls and fences it was like living in a fragrant, garden paradise.

But when Captain Keller was suddenly left a widower with two children he was grief stricken. Not even his young sons, James and Simpson, could console him and it seemed happiness would never come into his life again.

Some time later, however, when he met the beautiful, slim, fair-skinned Kate Adams, who had vivid blue eyes and golden hair, he fell in love with her. She was intelligent, charming, gentle and both of his sons adored her.

Arthur, a big, balding, but nevertheless rather handsome man was twenty years older than Kate and couldn't imagine that she would love him in return. Yet, not only did Kate love and want to marry him, she also loved his two boys.

Sure of rejection, it took a lot of courage for Arthur to propose to her and he could scarcely believe it when she accepted.

He wasn't very rich and Kate had come from an extremely wealthy home where she had led a pampered life. Nevertheless, once married, she proved to be the perfect wife and mother, always happy to help the servants around the house, cooking, gardening and doing the family sewing.

A short time after their marriage when Kate discovered she was going to have a baby the family was delighted. Even thirteen-year-old Simpson and James, aged nineteen, looked forward eagerly to the arrival of a new brother or sister.

Baby Helen Adams Keller was born on June 27th, 1880. She was a pretty little child with fair skin like her mother and a smattering of red-brown hair like her father, and it soon became apparent that she was also an exceptionally bright baby.

By the time she was eight months old she had begun to talk and could say 'How dee' and 'Tea' and her attempt at 'water' amused everyone when it always came out as 'wahwah'.

Without ever crawling or stumbling, at exactly one year old, she walked. This happened one day when she was sitting in her mother's lap being dried on a fluffy, white towel after her bath. Suddenly, she struggled from Kate's arms and set off at a trot on chubby little legs to catch a sunbeam shining on to the floor from the window.

By the time she was eighteen months old, Helen was very advanced — but then, early in the February of 1882, just a few months before her second birthday, illness struck.

At first it appeared to be a simple fever but then her temperature rose alarmingly and, at one stage, her life seemed in danger. Remember this was a hundred years ago. Her doctors were absolutely baffled and diagnosed the illness as acute congestion of the stomach and brain. Today's doctors recognise the complaint as Encephalitis — a form of meningitis with complications — and know how to treat it. At that time they didn't.

After some days, quite suddenly, the fever subsided and the Keller family and friends wept for joy; a joy that was sadly short lived.

When Helen began whimpering constantly and staring vacantly at the wall rather than turning her head towards them when they spoke everyone thought she was confused and perhaps a little afraid. After all, a baby wouldn't understand what illness was and why she had been feeling so wretched. But as the days passed she failed to respond to anyone or anything and when her little hands groped and clutched at the air, the terrible truth registered. The fever had left Helen both blind and deaf.

Maybe it was from weakness, they thought, and in a little time she would recover. But they were wrong. The light had gone out forever and with it went all the beautiful sights and sounds there are on God's earth. No more would she hear music, laughter, birdsong or the sweetness of her mother's voice.

Terrified and bewildered in her lonely, silent world, baby Helen wondered why it was always night, and day never dawned. She spent all her days either sitting in Kate's lap or, clinging tightly to her skirts, padding along behind her wherever she went.

Her parents and brothers were devastated. It was almost like losing her and yet she was still there in their midst. Trying to convey through touch that they were still there,

11

even if she couldn't see or hear them, they loved and cuddled her at every opportunity.

The fact that Helen was so young had mixed blessings. Although an older child would have remembered far more of the sights and sounds of the world around her, she would also have been acutely aware of all she'd lost. However, as all babies forget their earliest days, Helen would soon forget not only a time when she could see and hear but also *what* she had seen and heard.

For a while, tucked away in the recesses of her mind, lived vague memories of *green* fields, *blue* skies and *rainbow-hued* flowers but soon the colours faded.

The few words she had learned stayed with her a little longer. But as she couldn't hear her own voice, let alone anything else, there was nothing to associate them with and gradually they, too, were lost. The very last word she remembered was 'wahwah' until eventually even that was forgotten. The only natural sounds left were those of crying and laughter.

As the months went by Helen grew accustomed to her handicap. It was as though her life had never been any other way and, being a baby still, she didn't realize that she was different from those around her.

Even so, although blind and deaf, Helen was as mentally alert as ever. She was full of curiosity and, with her sense of touch enhanced through loss of sight and hearing, she took more notice than usual of everything around her. For ages she would examine and caress an ornament, toy, piece of clothing, animal, flower, absolutely anything until she knew everything about it and would recognise it the instant she came in contact with it again.

Maybe from pure instinct or because they were still locked away in her subconscious, she began using gestures to indicate what she wanted. A vigorous shake of her head meant 'No' a nod meant 'Yes'. A chewing motion meant she was hungry, and if accompanied by a forward and

12

backward movement of one hand against the other it meant she wanted bread and butter or a sandwich. Going towards the ice-box and shivering indicated that she wanted ice-cream. A push told someone to 'Go!'. A tug meant either 'Come!' or 'Give me your attention'. She referred to her father by going through the actions of putting on glasses; for *mother* she stroked her cheek while her father's sister, Aunt Ev, who lived with them, was indicated by piling her hair up at the back of her head. In all Helen perfected *sixty* different actions.

She could distinguish fabrics and knew if people were dressed to go out or were in the clothes they wore around the house. Vibrations reached her, telling her if someone was opening or closing doors; going up or down the stairs. She recognised footsteps and so knew whether they were approaching or leaving the room or the house. Departing guests were always given a 'farewell' wave. She could even *sense* when *something* special was happening, whether it was simply that guests were expected or that Christmas was approaching.

Feeling helpless in the situation, everyone overindulged the little girl and unwittingly did many of the wrong things. As she grew older she was treated more as a badly trained, untamed pet rather than as a human being and was taught none of the social graces, not even to use a knife and fork.

At the table she behaved like a little animal relying on instinct more than training. Plates were passed directly in front of her and halted while her fingers rummaged about in the food until she found some tasty morsel that appealed to her. Grabbing it she would cram it into her mouth then raid someone else's plate when it came within reach.

Although no one encouraged her to be independent in any way, her own nature and intellect spurred her on. Before she was five, she was able to help fold the clean laundry, pick out her own clothes and lay them to one side ready for the wardrobe or drawers. Other than that task, which was treated as a game, absolutely everything was done for her. She was downright spoiled and very soon became aware that she was never denied anything.

As she grew a little older the very thing her family had always dreaded finally happened. Helen began to realize that she was unlike everyone else and that there was something lacking in her existence.

She was curious about the way people often sat facing or stood close to each other. What were they doing? Sometimes when she clambered on to her mother's lap vibrations from Kate's body ran through her own. She would then place her hand to her mother's mouth and feel rapid movements. Sensing this was a form of communication Helen would open and close her own mouth in imitation. But when nothing happened and she gained no satisfaction from her efforts she would fly into a screaming tantrum and race from the room. Finding her old nurse, Viny, she'd scratch, thump and kick out at her and then cuddle up to kiss her by way of apology, only to repeat the attack the following day if the mood took her.

On other occasions, guided by the smell of various flowers growing in different parts of the garden or groping her way along the dark-green leathery leaves of the rigid, boxwood hedges skirting the garden paths, she would make her way to her favourite places. There she would sulk and, again depending on her mood, would either pummel or curl up with her doll to cry out her desperate longings. She adored Nancy, a rag-doll with brown, glass-bead eyes and a red-and-white check gingham dress; all of which Helen knew nothing — not even that it was a doll let alone that her name was Nancy. But then Helen didn't know that *she* was *Helen*.

One of her special haunts was an old, disused summer-house at the end of the garden near the orchard. Here she would caress the tendrils of weeping vines or the fragile petals of sweet-smelling blossoms and weep with exasperation at all she yearned for so much – yet not knowing what it was she wanted.

In 1886 when Helen was six her mother had another baby; a blue-eyed, fair-haired little girl whom they called Mildred. All the family celebrated — except Helen. Of course, she didn't understand that she had a baby sister or even know what a baby was, so Mildred's arrival came as a terrible shock to Helen and was bitterly resented. No longer did she occupy everyone's sole attention and quite often when she went to climb onto her mother's lap, there was 'something' already there. Furious with jealousy, she sometimes tried to claw the intruder from Kate's arms. Out of pure frustration she would scream and throw things, often breaking valuable ornaments and toys.

Even without temper Helen invariably broke things as her hands sought employment. As she had never been taught how to create anything, her only sense of achievement was in destruction thereby proving she had the power to create something by reducing the whole to many fragments.

In those moments, the family was filled with pity and felt so helpless. With her brothers being much older than herself, Helen had never been taught to share people or possessions with another child. Now she felt pushed out and had no way of knowing she was loved as much as ever. Even with a younger child, whom he loved dearly, in the house, Arthur, a keen gardener, always made sure it was his little Helen who got the first crop of luscious strawberries and grapes and the juiciest water-melon. It was Helen he took round the orchard and hoisted shoulder high to feel the first of the season's shiny, round apples; the rough peel of oddly shaped pears and firm, fluffy peaches. It was Helen he carried round the farm, lifting her up to pat and stroke the horses and cows.

She never failed to be fascinated by her father's actions when he sat reading newspapers in his study or was surrounded by manuscripts for editing. Sometimes, when he'd finished, she would climb into his chair, put on his glasses and hold the papers close to her face in an attempt to discover why he did it.

Next to her parents and brothers, the person Helen loved most was Aunty Ev. Nothing was too much trouble for Evelyn Keller, not even in the middle of one night when Helen went to her room and almost dragged her out of bed because she believed it was morning. Patient as ever, Evelyn got up, washed and dressed then helped Helen to wash and dress before taking her downstairs where she cooked breakfast for them both, thus starting her day at 2 o'clock in the morning.

Helen's only child companion was the cook's daughter, Martha Washington. Although they were very close friends and Martha was slightly older, Helen bullied her terribly, but the little negro girl never complained and seemed to understand her more than most. It was as though they had discovered some form of communication; one which often got them into trouble.

Full of mischief, they would creep into the kitchen when Martha's mother wasn't looking, steal her freshly baked cakes and sneak off to the summerhouse to eat them. Another day, after finding some scissors, they sat giggling on the verandah steps while cutting chunks out of each other's hair.

One day when she was alone in the kitchen and Martha wasn't there to help, Helen accidentally spilled a glass of water over her apron and took it off to dry it by the fire. Not really knowing what fire was or how to dry the garment, she threw it on the hot ashes. Immediately it burst into flames setting her clothes and hair alight. Her screams brought Viny racing to her side to quickly throw a blanket over her and douse the flames, but by then Helen's arms were scorched and part of her long hair had gone. Still, her life had been saved, but it was a dreadful experience for everyone and especially for herself. She didn't understand what had happened, only that her arms hurt terribly. For a while after that she was subdued but no sooner were her burns healed than she was up to her old tricks again.

On a day when all the servants were out of the house she locked her mother in the pantry. Sitting on the verandah steps she laughed and laughed as she felt the vibrations of Kate pounding on the pantry door and calling for help. It was three hours before she was released.

Helen was actually banned from her grandmother's house after she entered the drawing-room wearing her grand-mother's red-flannel underwear, then, when chastised for it, viciously pinched the old lady and chased her from the room.

But the naughtiest episode of all was when she found her little sister had crawled into her doll's cradle and fallen asleep. Furious at the intrusion, Helen tipped the cradle upside down whereupon Mildred fell out and would have hit the floor with a thud had her mother not been close by to catch her.

That incident made the Kellers finally face the truth. Helen was quite out of control. Every day she grew more and more stubborn, belligerent and unruly. Of course, there was no way she could be punished or shown her parents' displeasure over her attack on the baby. But from then on she recognized a change in people's attitude towards her.

During the following weeks they noticed a change in Helen's attitude, too, as gradually she lost all interest in everything except food.

They couldn't know why, nor could she tell them that she had quite simply given in and accepted the lonely world in which she was trapped. There was no point in fighting it. There was no escape. It was easier to aimlessly wander about clutching her doll or to sit stroking the soft, warm thing that mostly lay on the verandah or walked beside her through the garden. This *thing*, although Helen couldn't

17

know it, was Bella, the fat, old black dog.

This great change in her was even more perturbing than her naughtiness but fortunately for the child, her family had the sense to know such behaviour could only mean she was very unhappy. Oh, if only something could be done for her, they thought, both for her own sake and for everyone else's. But what?

In the past they had considered private tuition but there was little hope anyone would come to such a lonely place as the Keller home, lying at the end of a dirt track some miles from the sleepy little town of Tuscumbia. And anyway, where would they find a governess to teach a blind, deaf child?

Just at this time when they were all trying to think of a solution, Kate, purely by providence, was reading Charles Dickens' 'American Notes'. These told of his visit to the United States, of all the people he had met and places he had seen. In particular, he mentioned the Perkins Institute in Boston, Massachusetts, where he met Laura Bridgeman, a deaf and blind woman. As a young girl, by using some special form of alphabet, she had been taught to read and write by a Dr Howe, the Institute director. Kate's heart leapt until she read more and discovered it had all happened fifty years earlier and that Dr Howe was now dead.

Still, she thought, even if they could have helped, it would mean plunging Helen into a strange environment — a thousand miles away — where no one understood her nor she them. And surely, if she was already unhappy in her own home in the midst of her own loving family such a move would make her even more miserable and invite further rebellion.

All the same, things couldn't be left as they were. In desperation they decided to consult yet another eye specialist of whom Arthur had recently heard. He was a Dr Chisholm who lived in Baltimore some nine hundred miles north east of Tuscumbia.

2

The search begins

Obviously the journey to Baltimore was going to take a long time and so, in case Helen proved too much of a handful for her parents, Aunt Ev went with them.

Helen, of course, had no idea where she was going or why. It wasn't her first train ride but it was the longest and also the first she had ever really taken notice of. And, perhaps because she was quite active, other travellers were more aware of her presence. They made a tremendous fuss patting her hands, stroking her head, giving her fruit and sweets.

Even the ticket-collector took her with him through the rows of carriages as he checked tickets. Returning her to her parents, he produced some sheets of card and taught her to use the ticket-punch then left it with her until more passengers boarded at the next station.

When this game began to pale Aunt Ev made a makeshift doll out of some towels. But when Helen explored her new toy and found it had no facial features, she distressed everyone by being more upset at the absence of eyes than anything else. She went to each person in the carriage pointing this out then dropped to her knees to grope amongst the luggage under the seat. Moments later she emerged with her aunt's cape which had a row of buttons down the front and, tugging two of them off, she made a sewing gesture which told Evelyn exactly what was required.

Following two days and nights aboard the train, the party had a welcome night's sleep in a Baltimore hotel. And after breakfast the next morning, full of apprehension, Arthur and Kate set off with Helen to see the ophthalmist.

Not unexpectedly, Dr Chisholm gave them no hope at all for any recovery. No surgery or medicine could restore their daughter's sight. They must accept the fact that she would always be blind as well as deaf. However, as Helen was obviously sound in mind, he felt certain she could be trained in some things and advised them to consult Dr Alexander Graham Bell, some fifty miles farther north, in Washington. When Dr Chisholm saw the looks of surprise on Mr and Mrs Keller's faces he explained that Dr Bell was not only the inventor of the telephone, for many years he had been concerned with teaching deaf people because his own wife was deaf.

Given fresh hope, the Kellers set off for Washington where they were greeted by Dr Bell, a kindly Scot, who sat Helen on his lap and gave her his pocket watch to play with. Familiar with the deaf, he understood all her gestures and, as with Martha Washington, they even seemed able to communicate a little. As Helen played, he observed her closely, noting how mentally bright she was and to her parents' surprise he compared Helen to Laura Bridgeman from the Perkins Institute — the very girl Kate had read about in Charles Dickens' report. But when she reminded him that Laura's tutor was dead, Dr Bell told her the present Director of Perkins, Mr Anagnos, was continuing to teach by Dr Howe's methods.

When her parents went on to describe the difficulties they had with Helen he agreed that it could make her worse if she were sent from home to live among strangers. What he had in mind was to find a suitable *private* tutor; one who would be happy living in a quiet place like Ivy Green away from the city bustle. He promised to write to the Institute immediately and the Kellers set off on their long homeward journey more optimistic than they had been in years. Helen travelled back not knowing where she had been or why. All she was aware of was the experiences of different movements, vibrations, people, beds, things to touch, smell and eat.

Meanwhile, Dr Graham Bell was busily occupied composing a letter to Mr Anagnos of the Perkins Institute.

Dr Samuel Gridley Howe was a typical example of nineteenth century philanthropy, dedicating his life to helping others. In his early years he travelled to Europe where he fought with the poet, Lord Byron, in the 1821 Greek revolution against the Turks. After spending seven years there he made his way home across Europe reaching France in 1830, just in time to fight in a minor revolution there.

On his return to America he was approached by a friend who had been instrumental in establishing a school for the blind on a site donated by a wealthy Bostonian, Colonel Thomas Perkins. When he said that Dr Howe would be the perfect Director, Howe wisely asked for time to think it over. Throughout the next few days, to ascertain the sort of problems he would encounter, he lived day and night with his eyes bandaged. At the end of the week, bruised and sore from falls and grazes, he accepted the post, but with one condition. He must return to Europe to study their advanced methods of teaching the blind, and to collect all the necessary literature. During that second tour of Europe he also managed to recruit two teachers of the blind for Perkins; one from Paris, the other from Edinburgh in Scotland.

Back in America and settled into his new post, he was approached by many wealthy Bostonians, all eager to help the deprived in any way they could, and that inspired him to establish a Massachusetts State Board of Charities.

In 1867 yet another revolution flared up between Greece and Turkey and, recalling his past involvement, Dr Howe collected funds for the refugees and travelled to Greece with money and provisions. Whilst there he met Michael Anagnostopoulos, a baker's son who was fighting on the same side as himself. Michael had been highly educated and was working as a journalist in Athens when the fighting broke out. When the revolution was over he wasn't welcomed back at his newspaper office and was reluctant to return to his small village where there would be no outlet for his intellect. As Dr Howe was in great need of a secretary at that time, he offered Michael the post which was enthusiastically accepted.

By the time he was ready to return to America, rather than employer and employee, the two had become firm friends and Michael agreed to go with him. On their arrival in America, Michael and Julia, Dr Howe's eldest daughter, fell in love and were soon married. Thus, the handsome young Greek, Michael Anagnostopoulos — now calling himself Anagnos — was not only Dr Howe's secretary and friend but also his son-in-law. The two worked closely for Perkins and as Gridley Howe grew older, Michael was given more and more responsibility. When Dr Howe died in 1876, his son-in-law was the obvious choice to take over as Director of the Institute, and so the Institute stayed 'in the family' and the Howe teaching methods were continued.

Now, as Michael Anagnos read Dr Bell's letter asking for information about a possible tutor for Helen Keller he wondered if this was the answer to Annie's prayers?

Joanna Mansfield Sullivan, known as Annie, had been born in Massachusetts on April 14th, 1866. Years earlier, her parents, a poor Irish Roman Catholic couple, had emigrated from Limerick in Southern Ireland during the potato famine. Their aim was to seek their fortune in America but while their relatives, who had emigrated at the same time, made good — one opening a shop, another becoming a tobacco farmer — Thomas and Alice Sullivan lived in extreme poverty. This was due entirely to

Thomas's behaviour as he was always causing trouble and getting into brawls. He was lazy, couldn't keep a job and whenever he did manage to earn some money it was all spent on alcohol even though he had a wife and five children to support.

Alice was a quiet, gentle woman who became badly crippled and barely able to walk after a bad fall when Annie, her first child, was only three. With faded hair and a lined face, Alice looked more like a little old woman than a girl still in her twenties. Living under constant threat of violence from her drunken husband, she painfully hobbled about on crutches trying to feed and care for her children. But when she died suddenly at the age of twenty-eight, only three of the children were still living.

To everyone's dismay, Thomas Sullivan refused to either care for them himself or provide for someone else to keep them. Mary, the youngest, a beautiful and healthy child, was adopted by Alice's sister. The other two children were less fortunate. No one wanted eight-year-old Annie, who was almost blind, or four-year-old Jimmy, who was crippled with a diseased hip and walked with a crutch.

In an attempt to help, their uncle, the tobacco famer, gave Thomas a cabin on his land to live in. Annie was to be his housekeeper. However, this soon proved impracticable. Their father was always beating them and they were always hungry, so Annie and her small brother were sent to Tewksbury Almshouse. This was supposed to be a charity home for the poor or orphaned but was, in fact, run on the lines of a Dickens' workhouse by harsh people incapable of either kindness or charity.

They were so badly treated, poorly clothed and fed that Annie's sight deteriorated even more, and Jimmy died within a matter of weeks.

Annie was devastated the morning she awoke to find his bed was empty, but she knew where to find him and crept into the 'dead house' to be near him. The people running the almshouse refused to send for a priest; they placed the small boy's body in the ground without burial service, or even a prayer.

Annie was inconsolable and never forgot or forgave them. From then on all she cared about was getting out of Tewksbury before her own life ebbed away — but it was to take a further four years before she attained her freedom.

That came about when Dr Howe, as Chairman of the Massachusetts State Board of Charities, decided to hold an enquiry after receiving complaints from the public about the conditions and high death rate at Tewksbury.

During a visit of investigators, one inmate — No 985, Annie Sullivan, by then aged fourteen — suddenly broke loose from the other inmates and ran towards the group crying, 'Mr Sanborn. Mr Sanborn. Please take me away from here'.

Stopped in their tracks, the inspection team turned to look at her and their leader asked, 'What is the matter with you, child?'

'I'm almost blind, sir, but I want to go to school,' she said.

Without a word, the group walked on leaving Annie to stare after them while the other inmates jeered at her boldness. But within half an hour the matron came to say she would soon be leaving the almshouse to go to school.

Wearing a faded red calico dress, black cotton socks and shabby black shoes, Annie arrived at the Perkins Institute for the Blind in Boston, Massachusetts, on October 7th, 1880 — exactly three months after Helen Keller was born. With her only other possessions, a blue, coarse cotton dress and a pair of black cotton socks, tucked under her arm in a newspaper, she was a picture of poverty and misery.

The Perkins Institute, whose pupils came from wealthy, cultured families, was a totally different experience from anything she'd ever known. She had had no education whatsoever and could neither read nor write, not even her own name. And as her first years had been spent in rough conditions, Annie had no idea of how to behave in polite Boston society.

Eager to acquaint themselves with the latest pupil, the girls gathered round her and, although they were blind, they soon realized from the feel of her bony body, the poor condition of her hair and the rough texture of her clothes that she was different from themselves.

When she unpacked her pathetic bundle, the catty ones demanded to know why she had so few clothes and no coat or even a toothbrush. Sneeringly they asked, 'Even if you are poor, why didn't your mother *make* you some clothes?'

'My mother's dead and so is my little brother,' Annie snapped before flouncing from the dormitory leaving the girls whispering and giggling.

It was the matron, Mrs Hopkins, a motherly widow who had lost her own daughter, who came to Annie's rescue. That first night she lent her a nightdress to sleep in and promised to find her some other clothes. Still, despite that show of kindness, Annie cried herself to sleep on that night, and on every other night during that first week.

Her ignorance and bad table manners were made fun of and, unwilling to accept that not all the girls at Perkins were so unkind, she was hostile to everyone.

Coming from the poorhouse — a fact she determined the other girls must never know — she was so ashamed of her lowly origins and upset at the way she was being treated that pride forced her to be unruly and rebellious.

Annie became deliberately dirty and adamantly refused to do anything she was told. She would verbally and physically attack everybody — often the very people who were being kind and trying to help her, and that included the teachers. Sadly, in her attempt to get even with her tormentors, she made herself all the more miserable. Fortunately though, unlike Tewksbury, Perkins was run by truly charitable people. She was given new clothes and, although it hurt her dignity to be put amongst the youngest children, she was taught to read and write and soon her natural intelligence began to show through.

Eventually, after much affection and coaxing, she settled down, and by choosing her friends carefully, she realized they weren't all her enemies. While she was at Perkins, the Massachusetts State Board of Charities paid for her to have two eye operations which greatly improved her sight. Full of gratitude for this and always remembering Jimmy, she started to help the children who had handicaps other than blindness or those who were slow to learn. Very soon it became clear that Annie Sullivan wasn't at all the little ogre she'd first pretended to be and instead she became the most popular girl at the Institute.

One of her closest friends was Laura Bridgeman, about whom Kate Keller had read in Charles Dickens' report. Laura, by then in her fifties, had been blind and deaf following an attack of scarlet fever when she was two. Scarlet Fever was a very serious illness in those days. When she was seven, Dr Howe heard of her from a friend and called on her parents with a view to bringing her to Perkins.

It was his fist encounter with someone suffering from both afflications and he was determined the child should grow up to be self sufficient rather than totally dependent on others. First, he began teaching her the names of objects by pasting papers on everything with their names spelled out in raised letters. Later, she was taught to read all sorts of things by the same method and then she progressed to writing. Soon after arriving at Perkins, a new alphabet for the blind was invented which consisited of spelling out words into the palm of the deaf/blind person's hand. But in addition to all that, Laura was taught to be more independent than her parents had ever permitted. She could care for her clothes and knew how to braid her

26

golden hair and coil it round her head. She also learned to knit and sew.

All of this was considered remarkable, and yet Laura was really only *half* educated. She knew very little of mathematics, nature, geography, science or the arts but had been taught English in its perfect grammatical form so that when she *spoke* it was pure text-book language. This made her conversation so unnatural that it was like that of a foreigner who wasn't too familiar with English.

She never ventured outside the Institute grounds except to visit her parents and was always happy to return to Perkins, the one place she felt secure. Still, along with many others, including Charles Dickens, Annie Sullivan was overawed when she met her.

Mrs Hopkins, the Institute matron, was like a mother to Annie. Right from the beginning she had been very sympathetic to the little waif and seemed to understand that her rebellious behaviour came from injured pride. Never having recovered from losing her own daughter, Florence, she all but adopted Annie. It was as though they needed each other.

Sophie Hopkins lived in at Perkins but her home was at Brewster on the Cape Cod peninsula a few miles out of Boston and, at holiday time, to Annie's delight she was invited to stay there. When Annie first saw Brewster she could scarcely believe there were such places on earth. All her years had been spent in the city and this was totally different; a lovely little fishing village where green fields lay on either side of sandy roads. Roads led to rows of cosy cottages that looked out to the sea where, even with Annie's dim eyes, fishing boats could be seen bobbing about off-shore. There were sandy beaches and little coves to explore and the people were warm hearted and friendly.

Holiday after holiday Annie went there; she had never known such happiness. But as she grew older an awful fear took hold of her. Someday she would have to leave the Institute and go out into the world to earn her own living.

The years crept by without her noticing and suddenly it was 1886. She had been at Perkins for six years. Now she was twenty and it was time for her graduation. As proof of all she'd achieved, Mr Anagnos chose her to make the valedictory speech that year which, of course, was a great honour, but it was a miserable time for Annie.

For the big day, Mrs Hopkins made her a beautiful dress in frothy, white muslin with lace ruffles and pearl buttons. After helping to pile up her long, black, curly hair into ringlets she then brought out of tissue wraps the pink satin sash her own daughter, Florence, had worn for her graduation day. Annie was so proud she thought her heart would burst.

Just before she stepped on to the platform, her favourite teacher, Miss Moore, came forward to pin a spray of pink rosebuds on to her dress and then leant forward to kiss her cheek, which was wet with tears. In the very moment she should have been at her happiest, Annie was desperately sad. Others waited with longing for that important day in their lives, but they were going home to their families. Annie had no one and leaving Perkins would be like being sent away from home — the only real home she could remember.

Nevertheless, as she heard Mr Anagnos annouce her name, she put on a brave smile and made the best leaving speech the Institute had ever heard. Praise poured on her from everyone. For a short time afterwards she stood still while the other girls crowded round to 'see' her; feeling at her flimsy dress and soft white satin slippers. Smelling the flowers and patting her new 'grown up' hairstyle.

But back in her room as she unpinned the rose corsage and took off the pink sash, taking care not to snag the smooth satin with her nails, the sadness swept over her again. Quickly she brushed away a tear and forced herself to think of her forthcoming holiday at Brewster with Mrs Hopkins. There would be time for worry afterwards, she told herself. But she wasn't really convinced.

It was while she was at Brewster that summer that she received the letter from Michael Anagnos telling her of the Kellers' visit to Dr Bell. Of how he had recommended Perkins as the solution to their problems and would she be interested in the appointment?

Annie stared at the letter. He couldn't mean her. Hadn't she once said, 'I would rather wash dishes than be a teacher.' Still, there were the words staring right back at her from the page. When Mrs Hopkins read it she pointed out what a good opportunity it was — probably the best she would ever have — and advised Annie to end her holiday and return to Boston to get more details.

At first she begged Mr Anagnos to try to find her work in Boston, but he shared the matron's opinion and Annie reluctantly agreed with him. This didn't mean, though, that she was about to collect her belongings and embark on the 1,000-mile trip to Alabama. Months of preparation lay ahead with no promise made to the Kellers other than that a *possible* candidate had been found.

Every day was spent studying till her head ached, she felt sick and her weak eyes watered and smarted. The whole of Laura Bridgeman's case history needed to be read along with all the relevant reports made by Dr Howe. She read and digested every book she could find on the education of the blind, the deaf and what — through ignorance of that condition — was often considered 'dumb'. Most of the books covered only one or other of the afflictions as education of the deaf/blind was an entirely new concept. At the end of a long, weary day she would stop and ponder on all that was expected of her. With only the smattering of teaching experience she had gained at Perkins, she had absolutely no experience of coping with Helen Keller's problems. She felt so inadequate and it was only the exciting challenge that spurred her on.

Finally, in January the following year, after seven months' hard work, Mr Anagnos felt she was reasonably qualified and wrote to the Kellers informing them that a suitable governess had been found. She was a gentlewoman of great intelligence who was thought very highly of at the Perkins Institute.

This description hardly applied to the dirty, disobedient, naughty little rascal he had taken in from Tewksbury six years earlier. He made no reference at all to her poor sight or that she had just recently undergone yet another eye operation.

Kate and Arthur were so delighted at the news that they failed to notice that he'd given no information regarding the lady's formal qualifications. All they knew was that she would be arriving in Tuscumbia, on March 1st, 1887.

With a small group of friends, Michael Anagnos accompanied Annie to the railway station in Boston to see her off. There were good wishes and smiles mingled with salty tears which hurt Annie's eyes yet, by then, she was starting to feel excited about the adventure she was facing.

Once the train started, though, the excitement suddenly left her to be replaced by deep depression. She was leaving everything and everyone she knew and held dear for an unknown place 1,000 miles away among total strangers to become governess to a handicapped child she had never seen. Whatever had she let herself be talked into? Why, only two decades ago, the North and South had been at war with each other, and hadn't Captain Arthur Keller been a Captain in the Confederate Army? And from the day General Lee surrendered his forces to General Grant, the Union leader, hadn't many southerners carried on the war in their hearts? What if they treated her as 'one of the enemy'?

Her doubts were interrupted by the guard coming to

check passengers' tickets. Then, as he handed Annie's back, he told her that they had been made out wrongly. This meant she would have to change trains so many times that her journey would take all of three days. Utterly dejected she broke down and cried causing the guard to be so upset he put his arms about her shoulders and asked if she was on her way to a funeral. When she said 'No' but continued to cry he gave her a bag of peppermints to cheer her up. Annie had to smile at his concern and though her tears cleared up how she wished she could turn the train round and return to Boston. Better still if she could turn back time by seven months.

3

'Teacher'

For several days an air of anticipation had hung over the
Kellers' house and conveyed itself to Helen. Everybody had
been rushing about; servants cleaning, her mother fussing
from room to room. Helen recognized the activities usually
associated with the imminent arrival of guests. She also
sensed this was no ordinary guest and that something
special was about to happen.

Her mother kept going off with her brother, James, in
the carriage and each time they returned Helen sensed they
were disappointed about something.

Then, on one occasion as the carriage vibrations reached
her, her father and younger brother, Simon, suddenly got
up from their chairs and hurried out to meet it. This hadn't
happened on previous occasions and Helen knew whatever
was expected to happen had happened. Following them
through the door and on to the verandah she stood, her
vacant eyes staring into the unknown.

First James came up the path followed by her mother.
When they reached her they halted. Different vibrations
came from the garden path in front of the house. She knew
a stranger was approaching. Helen could neither see the
newcomer nor ask who it was, but she was filled with
curiosity and felt slightly afraid as a strained atmosphere
slowly built up all around her. This was caused by Arthur
Keller's attitude as he surveyed the young woman who had
supposedly come to his daughter's aid. And the look of utter

dismay on his face caused everyone to shuffle their feet in embarrassment.

At the station Annie had noticed that Kate Keller was only about eight years older than herself, and her step-son about her own age. This immediately created a panic in her. How could her inexperience be of any use if such young and able people were unable to help the child? Was there something she hadn't been told? Was the child simple-minded? Was she frail and delicate?

Now, as she peered through her dim eyes and saw the Captain's reaction together with that of Simon's, a boy in his early teens who looked downright worried, her doubts increased.

Noting the lack of movement and aware of the growing tension, Helen, in a desperate, heartrending gesture, appealed for an explanation by holding out her small hand towards where she thought Kate was standing. In the next moment, instead of her mother's familiar touch, she felt the stranger grip her hand tightly then sweep her up in her arms in a warm embrace.

It had been a desperate and spontaneous move on Annie's part, as much to stop the burning, stinging tears from falling as in thankfulness when she first saw Helen.

Familiar with reticence in blind children towards strangers, Annie was surprised to find herself holding a bold bundle of inquisitive energy that was eagerly feeling her face, tracing each feature and stroking her hair. Struggling to be put down Helen ran her hands over Annie's clothes and stopped abruptly as her fingers encountered the tapestry handbag slung over her arm. For a moment she explored the clasp but when it failed to snap open she trailed her fingers all round the bag until she found the lock. Holding her hand up to Annie, she pressed her finger and thumb together as though holding a key and began turning her hand backwards and forwards. No one could possibly mistake her meaning and Annie let out a gasp of astonishment as Kate explained that Helen was hoping to find sweets in the bag.

'Oh, what an intelligent girl she is,' Annie exclaimed.

'Do you really think so?' asked Kate.

When Annie confirmed that she did, the relief in Captain and Mrs Keller made them forget how unsuitable she looked for the job, and they ushered her into the house.

After the servants had carried her case and large trunk into the hall, Annie took Helen's hand and placed it on the trunk. Then taking her other hand and pressing it against her face she made a chewing motion. Immediately Helen's face broke into a wide grin and again her mother explained that she thought it contained sweets.

'Well, it does,' said Annie, and with those words little Helen Keller's life changed and her world began to expand.

Annie had secretly dreaded meeting the child for fear she was a feeble minded, helpless invalid in which case she wouldn't have known how to treat her. Instead, she was mentally as bright as a button with none of the nervous twitches blind children often have. Granted, at first sight her face appeared inanimate, expressionless as though there was no life there, but that wasn't uncommon in the blind and deaf. She had a strong body, sturdy limbs, a mass of brown, wavy hair, a wonderful smile and a face like an angel — albeit a dirty angel. Despite having an obviously loving, caring family, her own nurse and servants, Annie was amazed at Helen's unkempt appearance. Her hair was a tangled mess. Her hands and face grimy. Her pink dress and white apron, apart from being covered in stains, were downright filthy.

This was a direct result of wandering around the farm or from playing with Martha in the garden, scrambling through hedges and rolling about on the lawn with Bella. And as she knew no table manners, every meal of the day saw food and drink spilled down her clothes which she refused to change. Any attempt to clean her up and comb her hair invited a frightening display of temper. Only on getting up in the morning or going to bed at night would Helen agree to being washed and having her hair combed. And it was only after getting undressed for bed that her clothes could be taken away for laundering. Of course, this was a side of the little girl's nature Annie knew nothing about — but she was soon to learn.

Once her luggage was taken up to her bedroom, Annie proceeded to unpack with Helen insisting on examining every item. Soon, from amongst her clothes, Annie brought out a package wrapped in tissue paper and after carefully unwrapping it she handed it to Helen. It was a present the blind children at the Institute had bought out of their combined pocket-money; an expensive china doll whose beautiful clothes had been lovingly sewn and knitted by Laura Bridgeman.

Eagerly, Helen took it and hugged it close. Then, gently taking her little hand in one of hers, with the index finger of the other hand, Annie traced out on the child's upturned palm the word d-o-l-l.

Helen's brow furrowed as she tried to reason out what Annie was doing. Intending to repeat the experiment, Annie took the doll from her again whereupon to her horror she released a torrent of screams, kicks and scratches.

Quickly she gave it back to Helen, and waited until she had calmed down, then once more she traced the word d-o-l-l in her hand. After a moment's hesitation, without actually taking it from Helen, she slightly eased the doll away, quickly thrust it back then spelled out the word again. Next she picked up Helen's old doll, Nancy, and repeated the lesson.

This time, thinking it was a game, Helen smiled, took Annie's hand in hers and, without having the slightest idea of what it meant, spelled out precisely with her grubby finger the word d-o-l-l.

Annie's red-rimmed eyes opened wide with surprise. Her

35

experiment had worked. Calling for one of the servants she asked her to go down to the kitchen for a small cake by way of reward. When the cake arrived, she placed it into Helen's hand and taking her other hand spelled out c-a-k-e. Again the child showed interest but Annie had learned her lesson too. When she saw how greedily Helen crammed the cake into her mouth she didn't dare take it from her while she spelled the word out again for fear of being savagely bitten.

Later, seated next to her at the dinner table, she was sickened at the way the little girl ate and was even more horrified at her family's acceptance of such appalling behaviour.

That night she lay awake for hours, her mind full of doubts. She realized it was out of misguided love that Helen was so untrained in even basic manners. But how could the people who loved her allow her to act like that? And what right had she, a newcomer, a total stranger, to tell them they were wrong? Yet of one thing she was certain. Although Helen Keller showed much promise, if Annie Sullivan was to stay at Ivy Green things must change. Helen must be taught and if gentleness and kindness didn't work then firmness, even harshness, must be tried.

Next morning Annie steeled herself to face the disgusting spectacle of the breakfast-table and noticed how James grimaced as his plate was raided. So there was one person in the family who shared her views, she thought.

Instead of lessons Annie decided to spend that day observing Helen closely to discover exactly what sort of child she was. By evening she was completely astounded at her range of activities.

Due partly to over-protective parents and to the child's own nature, plus her misfortune, it was usual for blind children to lack confidence in themselves and be timid. They rarely ventured far from one place, wanting only to be close to those people they were dependent on, but Helen Keller showed none of those traits.

Without her knowing, Annie followed as she left the house, walked purposefully down the wooden verandah steps and set off at speed along one of the paths. Keeping her distance lest the vibration of her footsteps betray her presence, Annie followed her to the stables where she fearlessly patted the horses then went on to the cowshed where the milkers were at work. Standing much too close to one cow she had her face swished by its tail but brushing it aside with a laugh she stood her ground.

Minutes later, with Annie still in pursuit, she left the farm buildings and ran along a different path where she found Martha Washington. As the two children greeted each other in their own peculiar fashion Annie signalled to Martha not to let Helen know she was there. When she knelt down, cupped her hands and placed them on the ground Annie was filled with curiosity.

'Whatever is she doing?' she asked.

Martha explained, 'She wants to collect the eggs.'

Off they all went to the hen coops where the girls gathered the eggs and Annie burst out laughing when she realized that Helen was insisting on carrying them back to the house herself in case Martha dropped them.

After Helen placed the eggs in a bowl in the kitchen Annie stepped forward, took her hand and led her upstairs to what had been designated as the schoolroom. There, she produced a set of 'sewing cards' with holes in them outlining the forms of animals, shapes and words. After letting her feel them for a while she threaded a broad needle with thick yarn, placed it in Helen's hand then took her other hand to instruct her on how to push the needle into one hole and out the other.

The child instantly took to this latest game — but ironically, the first word was 'card'. Annie didn't give a thought to it but no sooner had Helen sewn the letters 'c' and 'a' when she recognized the symbols. Making a chewing motion with her jaws she threw down the sewing and pushed Annie towards the door. How she laughed. Helen obviously remembered that after making those signs the previous night she had been given cake. Annie hadn't the heart to resist and sent to the kitchen for the expected reward. With that Helen happily resumed her 'game' and was so successful that Annie took the work down to the drawing-room for her parents' inspection. They were amazed, particularly when told that was only the beginning. Annie had already deduced that her pupil was not only capable of learning language but all the subjects a child would normally learn in school.

Until then, out of exasperation and frustration, Helen had destroyed most things. Her hands needed employment but because she was never taught to do anything creative her only sense of achievement was in breaking or destroying something. In that way it was within her power to create many fragments out of one whole.

Yet, although she had made such a good start, the weeks ahead weren't going to be easy for any of them. After the first week when she knew them better and was feeling more sure of herself Annie decided to put her position to the test.

They were all seated at table one morning being served breakfast with Helen as usual groping in the plates for food. But as Annie's plate came towards her and Helen plunged her hands into it, Annie firmly removed them. Again the little hands went in search of something and again Annie moved them away. This time Helen pinched her arm whereupon Annie gave her a sharp slap causing the family to gasp in shocked disbelief.

Helen made a terrible scene lying on the floor kicking and screaming. She tugged at the legs to pull Annie's chair from under her while her parents and brothers looked on in bewilderment. Annie meanwhile calmly sat eating her breakfast without glancing up from her plate. Twice Kate made a move towards the hysterical child but somehow sensed that Miss Sullivan wouldn't approve. After some minutes, the family got up from their breakfast and left the room. Determined not to be intimidated by the child or humbled by her family, Annie continued to eat.

After a few minutes when her fury was spent, Helen got up and sidled round to find out what Annie was doing. On discovering she was eating she made another grab at the plate and was once more firmly rejected. Desperate for sympathy she ran to the other chairs only to find them all empty. Finally admitting defeat she sat in her own chair and began to eat — with her fingers. Annie took a spoon and placed it in her hand. Smash it went to the floor. Picking it up, Annie spooned some food on to it before handing it back to Helen. Smash to the floor again, this time with food splattering over the carpet. It took half an hour to get Helen to accept that she either ate with a spoon or went hungry. Another tiresome hour was spent persuading her to fold her napkin before she could leave the table. By then they were both weary of each other and when Annie finally opened the door Helen fled towards the verandah as though Satan himself were at her heels. Annie raced in the opposite direction and went upstairs to fling herself on her bed and cry herself to sleep.

That evening before dinner, she had a serious talk with Helen's parents. If any progress was to be made she must be allowed to do it in her own way without interference. She didn't want to be hard on the child but already it was too late to teach her in a gentle manner. Breakfast had proven that only because she was hungry had she complied with Annie's wishes. And if that was the only way she could learn then so be it. It was going to be painful and unpleasant for everybody with ugly screaming, fighting scenes and while Annie was prepared to put up with that Helen's parents evidently weren't. Hadn't they gone without breakfast that morning for that very reason?

In their hearts they knew Annie was right and asked what she had in mind. When she said it was to take Helen away

39

from Ivy Green for a while they were appalled and reminded her they had hired a governess to prevent her from having to leave home.

'Oh, not far,' she said. 'Maybe rent a little house in the village.'

Then Arthur Keller remembered the old summerhouse at the far end of the orchard. There, Helen wouldn't actually be leaving home yet she wouldn't be in the house either. However, when Annie made him promise not to come near the place he didn't think it such a good idea after all. It was his sister who persuaded him after getting Annie to 'let him come by each day and peep in at the window without Helen knowing'.

Helen knew the summerhouse well and at the first opportunity would make her escape, so they changed all the curtains and furniture. On the morning they moved in, Annie and Percy, one of the servant boys, took her for a long walk through the woods surrounding Ivy Green. It was an area Helen didn't know but which led indirectly to the summerhouse. Consequently, she had no idea of where she was.

The temporary home was quite large yet consisted of only one room where Annie was determined they would live, eat, sleep and wash until Helen had been turned from a vicious, selfish little savage into a civilized human being. And she, more than anyone, hoped it wouldn't take long.

4

In search of knowledge

All their food would be delivered from the big house. Laundry would be collected and delivered back to them. Percy would do the dusting, sweeping and dish-washing leaving Annie to devote all her time to her pupil.

At first Helen was curious about her new surroundings and explored every angle of the room. If its shape seemed familiar, the strange furniture and curtains, together with a bed that had no place in a summerhouse, convinced her she was in a strange place. It was only as the day wore on and their meals were being eaten there that she showed alarm. Why weren't they going home? Where was her mother? Often she touched her cheek and ran to the door as though she expected Kate. When she didn't arrive, Helen heaved a big sigh and went to sit down again as though waiting . . . waiting.

When night came and Annie began getting her ready for bed, Helen put up a terrific struggle, fighting, kicking, biting, screaming and scratching. Suddenly her clenched fists landed an almighty blow which cracked two of Annie's front teeth and blacked her eye. Little Percy scuttered to his bed in the corner and nothing could induce him to venture out while the storm was raging. After *two hours* of violence, Helen was so worn out that Annie was able to undress her and put her to bed. But when she felt Annie get in beside her she let out a shriek and bolted from the bed. Again Annie tussled with her until finally she gave in

41

but lay as far from Annie as possible without dropping off the edge.

Helen awoke early the next morning and leapt from the bed to fumble her way around the strange environment, panic increasing with every second. For a moment Annie watched and could have wept for her. All her short life she had been cosseted and permitted to do excactly as she liked. And now, the very person most intent on helping her was forced into being downright brutal. Still, she reasoned, firmness would team with compassion, admonishment with love, but oh, Annie thought, if only I could make her understand why.

Still tired from the previous night's battle she dragged herself from the bed and patted the tender bruises on her mouth and her eye as she made her way to where Helen had slumped, weeping in utter dejection.

As soon as she felt Annie's reassuring presence beside her, Helen clung to her for an instant but then, gathering all her strength, pushed her away. Percy went out to sweep the path and wait for breakfast to be delivered while Annie got washed and dressed. Helen remained motionless on the floor until Annie indicated it was time for her to wash and dress. This she adamantly refused to do. When breakfast arrived and she smelled the delicious hot food, she followed her nose to the table but Annie took her hand and led her to the wash-bowl. Over and over this happened until she sank to the floor again and Annie left her there while she ate her own breakfast which was by then cold and barely palatable.

Just then Arthur Keller went to peep through the window and what a sorry sight met his eyes. The 'teacher' was tucking into her meal while his small daughter sat on the floor, crying and hugging Nancy. She was unwashed, undressed and her food lay untouched on the table. He was furious and stormed back to the house to relate his story to Kate and his sister, Ev.

'No child of mine shall be denied food,' he fumed. 'I've a mind to pack that young woman off back to Boston on the next train.'

Kate agreed with him until Evelyn reminded them that they had promised to leave Helen with Miss Sullivan at the summerhouse for a month yet this was only the first morning.

For the rest of that morning Helen played with her dolls, dressing and undressing them until she grew bored and flung them unlovingly into a corner. As the day wore on she assumed a similar attitude to the one that she had adopted after tipping Mildred out of the cot. Her family had abandoned her to the clutches of this stranger so she may as well obey her every command. There was no use in fighting.

This placid acceptance of her fate was the last thing Annie wanted. The child had a strong spirit which mustn't be broken under any circumstances. Whatever was she to do? Was there no way of breaking through into that silent, black world?

The first thing to establish was order — just as with the sewing cards, her life needed a pattern to work to. Until then, the only order she knew was mealtimes and bedtime. For the rest she was left merely to *kill* time. From now on she must learn to *use* it.

For a few days they continued with the sewing cards and then Annie introduced her to bead threading. First, she acquainted her with the broad needle and string with its bulky knot on the end to make her understand that they were much bigger than those for sewing cards. Next she brought out some assorted beads in wood and glass, and guiding Helen's hand, threaded two wooden beads followed by one glass; two wood and one glass.

Helen ran her fingers over them and when Annie was sure she knew the sequence, indicated that she was to thread them herself. Each time she made a mistake — one wood, one glass — Annie took them off the string and made her

43

do them again. It took a lot of patience from the teacher and even more from the pupil but then, suddenly, she started threading them in the right order and a beam spread across her face. It was the first time she'd smiled since leaving home.

The next day she was taught to crochet with some bright red wool — which, of course, Helen couldn't see. Crocheting was easy and by nightfall she'd made a chain which stretched halfway across the room. Now she actually laughed aloud. Annie was so pleased she put her arms around Helen and kissed her cheek and, for once, the little girl didn't protest.

Mealtimes were still battles but at least Helen had stopped trying to delve her hands into Annie's plate. Even so, although she would get a slap and have her food taken away, she persisted in throwing her napkin and spoon to the ground and eating with her fingers. Only from sheer hunger and as a result of Annie's perseverance would she concede. Then, after she'd eaten, there followed another tiresome episode to get her to fold her napkin.

Arthur Keller came regularly to peep through the window and each morning he saw an improvement in his child's appearance and attitude. The day he saw her sitting beside Annie, serenely crocheting, with her clothes, hands and face clean, her hair neatly combed and beribboned, he raced back to the house to tell Kate.

Helen was learning to spell more words every day although she had no idea what *words* were. And then one morning, two weeks after moving to the summerhouse, just when Annie was beginning to think she was the wrong teacher for Helen, there came the breakthrough she'd prayed for.

It was breakfast-time and Helen spelled out m-u-g which told Annie she wanted a drink. Annie poured some milk into the mug and spelled out m-i-l-k. But this proved too much for Helen and no matter how often Annie spelled m-i-l-k, Helen repeatedly spelled m-u-g.

After a moment's thought Annie led the child over to the wash-stand where the ewer was full of water and spelled w-a-t-e-r. Then she took her back to the table, poured some milk into the mug and spelled out m-i-l-k.

Eventually, Helen got so fed up she punched Annie and then ran to where her new doll sat on a chair. Picking it up, she dashed it to the floor where it shattered into dozens of pieces. Not sure if her efforts had worked she stooped to examine it and finding it broken, beamed with happiness. Then, defiantly, she took hold of shabby old Nancy and burying her face in the soft, rag body sobbed and cuddled her.

Annie kept her patience. She knew Helen was telling her that she loved Nancy but the new doll meant nothing to her because it was she who had given it to her. She couldn't be told that it had been a gift of love from all those other blind children, not yet anyway.

Then, in a flash, Annie realized it was she who was being stupid. Helen genuinely believed m-u-g represented cup, drink, water and milk.

Gently, she lifted Helen into her arms and carried her out of the summerhouse to the pump in the yard. By chance, Percy was drawing water and as the first trickle rose to the top and quickly developed into a steady flow, Annie thrust Helen's hand under it while into her other hand she spelled w-a-t-e-r. Next she thrust the mug into her hand and spelled m-u-g.

Following that she held Helen's hand under the pump while the mug filled up with water. Suddenly, as though a dark cloud had moved away from the sun, Helen's face lit up in awareness. In that moment she realized what Annie was doing. Hastily, her mind recalled how when the *thing* she'd just destroyed was first placed into her arms the newcomer had made movments on her hand. When she was given something to eat there were more signs. Then more

45

when she held a cup. Now they had changed again and yet, although they kept changing, many were repeated but in a different order.

What until then had been objects known only by touch, taste or smell were falling into their individual slots. She reasoned that everything must have its own signs — and yet, of course, she didn't even know the word *signs* or any other word for that matter. Yet, in a sense she did. *She simply didn't know they were words.*

Water or 'wahwah' had been the last word she'd ever spoken. Now it was that very same word that had awakened her mind. Like some wild thing let out of a cage she began dragging Annie after her, pointing at everything they passed, stopping to pick up others then holding out her hand for the signs to be made.

Annie could hardly keep up with her and her mind whirled as she spelled d-o-g; f-l-o-w-e-r; t-r-e-e; h-o-u-s-e. It was impossible for Helen's mind to absorb every word at once but now she knew everything had a name and that she was capable of learning them, on and on she went.

Exhausted but none the less excited, Annie allowed herself to be pulled, pushed and hurried along the path with each step taking her nearer to the big house.

Attracted by the commotion from outside Aunt Ev, Arthur and Kate came out on the verandah. In speechless astonishment they stood looking at the spectacle of Kate and Annie racing round like mad things until suddenly they understood what was happening.

When Helen realized she was in her own front garden and that her parents and Aunt Ev were there she ran, embraced them and then ran back to Annie who spelled out m-o-t-h-e-r, f-a-t-h-e-r, a-u-n-t.

They were overjoyed. 'She knows us. Our little girl knows who we are,' Kate cried.

But after watching her for a while they grew concerned about her getting over-excited and tiring herself out with her new discoveries. Could her mind withstand such a bombardment of information, they asked and insisted she stop and go inside to rest. This infuriated Helen and threatened to bring on one of her now almost forgotten tantrums so Annie quickly took her back to the summerhouse.

At last she knew what Annie was doing. What she had been trying to do all the time, and throughout the rest of the day she demanded to know what everything was. That evening as she was getting ready for bed she pointed to Annie who spelled out T-e-a-c-h-e-r, and from then on Helen called her by that name.

As they fell into bed thoroughly exhausted, Helen, to Annie's delight, snuggled up in her arms, kissed her and fell into a contented sleep.

The arrangement had been to stay at the summerhouse for one month but, once Helen knew where she was, there was little point in keeping her there. The next morning they packed and returned to Ivy Green with Helen demanding to know more names all the way along the path.

Poor Annie. Her eyes hurt constantly yet Helen must never know. Anyway, she was every bit as determined as her pupil that lessons go on. She had an earnest talk with Mr and Mrs Keller explaining that although she and Helen were living back at the house, her methods must still be observed. Also, they must not worry about their daughter's brain being overtaxed. Her mind was like a book filled with blank sheets of paper waiting to be written on.

That evening none of the family ate so intrigued were they by Helen. She arrived at the supper-table with freshly washed hands and face, put on her napkin and waited for her meal to be served. Two plates of delectable food wafted past her to be placed in front of her parents but she made no attempt to investigate. When the third plate was put down before her she reached for her spoon and began to eat in a manner they had never expected to see. At the end of supper, when one of the servants came to clear the table, Bella waddled into the room. Immediately, Helen knew she was there and ran to hug the fat old dog who had evidently missed her.

'She's trying to teach the dog to spell,' laughed James as his sister took Bella's paw in her own small hand and wrote d-o-g.

On the day following their return they were in the garden when Viny brought Mildred along. Now, thought Annie, is a good time to introduce Helen to her baby sister, who, until then, she had considered a rival. Annie encouraged her to feel the small body, stroke her hair and trace the dimples on the backs of her podgy hands. When she reached her mouth and realized she was smiling, Helen embraced and kissed her. More than that, she took hold of her hand and walked her round the garden all the time talking to her in her sign language. This, of course, made no impression on Mildred who chatted away in her own baby talk not knowing she couldn't be heard. In that moment Annie was more proud of turning Helen into a sweet, loving, civilized child than of all the academic achievements she may acquire in the future.

As she watched them Annie wondered how she could teach her to converse naturally rather than simply knowing isolated words. Laura Bridgeman had never accomplished the art. She had been so well tutored to use perfect grammar that quite often she hadn't made sense, as on the occasion she asked, 'Is it a derivative day?' Later, Annie learned that this was because she'd been told that 'rainy' was the derivative of 'rain'.

Watching Viny with Mildred, she pondered on how babies learn language. They are not taught isolated words. But as she sat there the answer was presented to her when Helen picked a flower for Mildred and Viny said, 'Go, take it to your mummy'. Without hesitating the baby toddled off along the path towards the house.

Of course! That was it! Viny hadn't said 'Flower. Mummy. House'. Babies are listening to their language from the day they're born. That's how they learn. From then on Annie spelled out whole phrases such as, T-h-i-s i-s a c-a-t. T-h-a-t i-s a d-o-g. H-e-r n-a-m-e i-s B-e-l-l-a.

During the following two weeks, along with the numerous nouns she'd already learned, Helen added a further 400 words to her vocabulary.

In fine weather they practically lived outside, their schoolroom consisting of soft cushions heaped into the forked branches of a huge tree. Annie was determined right from the start to abandon all idea of formal lessons. Helen may be almost seven years old, but in terms of scholarship she was a baby, and who would expect a baby to sit at a desk or table for long periods learning first one subject then another? No, she must learn naturally as she went along and with such an eager pupil asking endless questions, her knowledge would quickly grow.

Helen never stopped for a moment, spelling words so quickly that Annie could barely keep up with the answers. Gradually and unconsciously she absorbed other parts of grammar and was soon rapidly spelling out, W-h-a-t i-s . . . ? W-h-y i-s . . . ? H-o-w . . .? When . . . ? Where . . . ?

With each day that passed, Helen grew more pretty as her features became more animated. It was as if her ever-expanding mind and her soul glowed out from her face.

One day, she was curious to know why some plants grew up walls and fences. When Annie explained that they were creepers, Helen wanted to know 'What are creepers?' That led to a demonstration of creeping followed by walking, running, hopping, skipping.

Annie feared that the biggest hurdle was going to be teaching her the abstract. It was all very well putting labels on items that could be touched, tasted or smelled. But there were such things as love, colour, air and sky. Oh, how can she possibly comprehend all of that, she wondered?

It proved easier than Annie expected. One morning when Helen was threading her beads into a pattern she'd devised herself, she became confused and asked Annie what was the sequence. Without a thought Annie gave her the first inkling that there was more than material things in the world when she tapped Helen's forehead and spelled into her hand t-h-i-n-k.

Helen's brow furrowed. 'W-h-a-t i-s t-h-i-n-k . . . ?' she demanded to know.

Annie's heart sank. How ever was she going to explain this? To the best of her ability she wrote into Helen's hand that every living creature had a brain situated in their head and that everything she had ever learned was stored there. She explained that the very thing she was describing at that moment was going into storage to be called upon at any time.

Instantly Helen understood what Annie was saying and after a minute during which she consciously *thought*, she proceeded to thread the beads in the right sequence. From there it was easy for her to grasp that not everything in the world was tangible.

Her next discovery was size and emphasis. Some things were big; others small. Some were *very* big; some *very* small.

Within three months of Annie arriving, Helen had learned so many words it seemed appropriate that she should learn to read. Braille — the form of communication used by blind people — had only recently been invented and wasn't in common use at that time so Annie taught her to read by the method they used at Perkins. This was simply having words on a page printed in large, raised letters. To Helen, being able to read books was like stepping into another world; a world teeming with curiosities all of which needed explanation. What she did not know was that all her additional questions sapped her teacher's energy.

All the family learned the finger alphabet but Arthur

Keller never really grasped it. He would sit Helen on his lap and begin telling her a story but got into such a muddle that she would first start to titter and always ended up rocking with laughter. To see his daughter so happy pleased him more than anything and he would reflect on the past years of despair when no one could have dreamed he would ever be telling her a story — let alone one she often completed herself.

At the end of May, the beautiful balmy spring gave way to a stifling hot summer, and as June wore on Annie told Helen that she was nearing her seventh birthday. This took some explaining of years, months and weeks; it also introduced Helen to numerals. This prompted her to count every conceivable thing: fingers, toes, eyes, ears, beads, stairs, flowers, berries, railings, cutlery, crockery, even wall tiles. Up and down she raced in search of more quantities to be checked.

When one of the farm dogs produced a litter of five puppies she was taken to 'see' them but panicked as the puppies began feeding. Helen thought they were 'eating mother dog'. Then she wanted to know where the eggs were that they'd come out of, and that question led to her learning of the wonderful process of birth.

As the summer heat intensified everyone became alarmed at Helen's appearance. She was pale, thin and easily fatigued but persisted in work, work and yet more work, falling asleep in Annie's arms while still spelling out questions.

When it was suggested that all the work was making Helen ill, Annie argued that the weather was causing the problem. She, too, was thoroughly exhausted. The dry, airless conditions caused her eyes to sting and itch making them raw and red-rimmed, and, although happy in her work, she longed for the cooler air of Boston.

All the time she had been at Ivy Green, she had been writing to Mrs Hopkins and Mr Anagnos telling them of

Helen's progress. You should come to Alabama and see for yourself, she told the Institute Director. He wrote back suggesting she bring her prodigy north to see him and to be introduced to the children at Perkins.

Oh, if only I could, she thought, but put the notion firmly at the back of her mind — for then at least. Meanwhile, something needed doing to stop Helen from being so active.

She had read all her specially printed books. New ones were on order from Philadelphia but they took a long time to arrive. Maybe if she learned to write that would entail sitting quietly and conserving her energy, thought Annie. Thus she was introduced to pen and paper.

As with her reading, Annie didn't use the Braille alphabet but what were known as 'box letters'. They were raised letters on a board that could be placed under a sheet of paper and traced over with a stylus pen. Usually a rather slow process, it proved very easy for Helen who was already familiar with the Roman alphabet. After settling her down to pursue this new gentle activity Annie would have time to write letters to Sophie Hopkins and Michael Anagnos.

One day Helen was so quiet that Annie kept looking to see if she had fallen asleep at the table but she was concentrating on her work.

At the end of the session, Helen went to Annie and asked her to put on her coat. Annie asked why and looked at the piece of paper she'd had thrust into her hand. None of the letters was properly formed but she didn't say so. When she asked again why she must put on her coat, Helen explained that she had written a letter to her Uncle Frank, and wanted to post it.

'And what does the letter say?' asked Annie.

Uncle Frank. Much words. Puppy mother dog five. Baby cry. Hot. Helen walk — no. Strawberries very good. Frank come. Helen kiss Frank. Teacher put letter in.

There the letter ended because although she had been to the post-box many times with Annie she didn't know the name of it. Nevertheless, Annie wasn't going to disappoint her. She quickly wrote a note for Frank Keller telling him of Helen's attempt to send a letter, which she included along with its translation, and asked if he would please answer it.

That evening, the heat wave finally broke when the longed-for rain lashed down accompanied by a frightening thunderstorm. Helen couldn't hear the thunder crashing overhead nor could she see the lightning flashes but she *felt* the storm.

The next morning was much cooler and everything looked fresh, but the earth had been so parched that all signs of the torrential rain had gone. Helen was surprised and asked if the flowers and trees had drunk it all.

Every day, week and month that went by her knowledge grew and the more she learned, the more she was able to learn by her own ability, reasoning things out for herself. Sometimes, as with the flowers and trees drinking all the rain, she made wrong assumptions, but they were the same as those any seven year old makes.

With every letter to Mrs Hopkins and Mr Anagnos, Annie told them of each new accomplishment. Mr Anagnos was immensely proud that the pupil of one of Perkins' own graduates was progressing so well that he recorded it in the Institute Reports. Soon the press got hold of the story of little Helen Keller, and without her knowing, she became a national heroine with every American clamouring to hear of her latest achievements.

5

Filling the blank pages

Throughout her childhood Helen had travelled quite a lot with her parents, mostly to see different doctors, so she knew there was a world outside of Tuscumbia. And once she had learned to read she quickly discovered that there was a world outside of America as well.

'What are oceans and ships?' she asked. 'What are nations?' 'What is snow?' 'What are maps?'

To give her a practical demonstration, 'Teacher' took her for a stroll through the estate to a small inlet on the Tennessee River called Keller's Landing. It was a place to which Helen had never been and she was placed under strict promise never to go there unless accompanied by an adult. After letting her paddle in the water for a while, Annie collected some mud from the water's edge from which she made a model depicting mountains and valleys. Pouring water into the hollows, she made seas and rivers. Deserts were represented by handfuls of powdered dry mud from farther up the bank. When it was finished, Helen explored the miniature world with her sensitve fingers while Annie told her of far off lands with their different climates, flora and fauna; their peoples, languages, histories and cultures.

Another day they went to the zoo where she met some of the strange animals she'd either read or been told about. One evening she was taken to a circus where she rode on an elephant and was allowed to stroke some lion cubs.

Naturally, these activities increased Helen's curiosity and

she longed to travel and see all the wonders for herself.

By now, she always spoke of 'seeing' people and things and with her lively imagination she was almost correct because she was *seeing* with her mind. Wherever they went, riding in the carriage or walking, Annie described everything they passed. Consequently, Helen probably accumulated more information than other children her age who were left to see for themselves, and probably didn't bother to question what they saw. Maybe it was living in a black, soundless world with no distractions that increased her capacity to concentrate.

Eager to show off their now sociable child, the Kellers started paying more calls on friends and relatives and Helen revelled in it. Her new found self respect promoted such pride in her appearance it was difficult to believe she was the same scruffy, dirty child of a few months earlier. Putting on a hat she would stand posing in front of the mirror as though seeing herself.

On one occasion when they were going to pay a call after lunch she decided to get herself ready. First, she plastered her long, thick chestnut hair with her father's hair oil. This was followed by putting her mother's skin cream all over her face and then powdering over the whole lot before putting on her best hat and frock. When Kate and Annie saw her coming downstairs they laughed so much that they had to throw their arms around each other and hang on for support.

In August, Arthur took her to Huntsville, about seventy miles east of Tuscumbia, to visit his mother. Because of Helen's previous bad behaviour she had been banned from her grandmother's home, so father and daughter stayed in an hotel. People who hadn't already read about her in the newspapers were intrigued watching her communicating with her father and her teacher, and everybody lavished attention on her.

As each person introduced him or herself, Annie translated it to Helen who politely shook hands with them. The following morning, to their amazement, she remembered each individual by name.

Other children in the hotel were fascinated by her. When she began tapping her foot in time to the vibrating beat of some music, one little girl led her by the hand on to the floor where she taught her to dance the polka. A small boy introduced her to his pet rabbit and, in turn, Helen taught them the finger alphabet.

On the day of their visit, her grandmother didn't recognize her. The last time they met, Helen had been unruly, bad tempered, ill mannered and dirty. Now she saw a clean, smiling, pretty child in an immaculately white lawn dress. And not only that. Instead of a tangled mass, sticky from the breakfast marmalade she'd rubbed into it, her shiny, chestnut hair was adorned by a satin ribbon and hung in ringlets down her back. No matter how tired Helen was, before going to bed, she would insist that her hair be put into curl papers every night.

As Kate hadn't been able to go with them, Helen wrote giving all the news of relatives and friends in Huntsville.

helen will write mother letter. papa did give helen medicine mildred will sit in swing mildred will kiss helen teacher did give helen peach george is sick in bed george arm is hurt anna did give helen lemonade dog did stand up
conductor did punch ticket papa did give helen drink of water in car carlotta did give helen flowers anna will buy helen pretty new hat helen will hug and kiss mother helen will come home and mother does love helen
good-by

It was the first letter she had ever sent to her mother and the absence of capital letters and punctuation was irrelevant. Until a short time ago, her daughter didn't have a solitary word in her head and Kate treasured the letter for the precious manuscript it was.

That holiday was the happiest Arthur Keller had known since Helen was a baby. On the way home to Tuscumbia, to give her the sensation of climbing and thus help her understand what a mountain really was, Annie asked if they could take the route past Monte Sano — a well-known mountain in the area. Imagine their surprise when she later described Monte Sano to her mother as having 'cloud caps'. The sky had been a cloudless azure blue that day but her vivid imagination had painted its own picture.

When a letter came for Helen one day from James Adams, one of her uncles, Annie read and re-read it to her until she knew it by heart. But when she ran to show it to her mother, Bella and Mildred, the dog wasn't at all impressed and Mildred promptly grabbed it and chewed it up. Helen was so furious with her little sister she slapped her hands. Annie explained that the baby didn't know she was doing wrong. At this Helen was so full of remorse at losing her temper she promised to 'write baby a letter full of beautiful words for her to eat'.

She was writing letters daily now to her grandmother, aunts, uncles, cousins and Mr Anagnos, with each letter showing great improvement on the last. Almost without noticing she was mastering punctuation and capital letters. Her latest problem was that once the 'box letter' board was removed from under the paper, Helen couldn't read what she had written. Annie decided it was time to teach her Braille, and as this is almost like learning another language, it meant that by October, Helen, who had no language at all in March, was embarking on learning a second one.

As with everything else, she soon grasped the idea of translating the patterned spots into letters and words. Now she could write not only to Mr Anagnos at the Perkins Institute but also to the students. Regarding them, Helen simply could not comprehend that they could be blind without also being deaf.

When they got her first letter they were delighted, as was Laura Bridgeman who already knew about her from Annie's letters.

Annie had asked Mr Anagnos to write and persuade Helen's parents to let her go to Boston for a few weeks to meet other blind children. As well as for her own sake, it would boost their morale if they met someone as bright, confident and capable as seven-year-old Helen Keller.

But, before then, Christmas was approaching fast. On every previous occasion over the past seven years the fesitivites had been ruined with tantrums. That year Helen would join in the celebrations and everyone revelled in the exciting preparations.

Being able to talk to her, everybody teased her by pretending to write into her hand what she would be getting — only to stop abruptly as though they'd suddenly remembered that she mustn't be told.

And it pleased them immensely when she proved to have a great sense of humour by doing precisely the same to them. For weeks, she and 'Teacher' had been buying and making presents for everybody and if Helen could be teased then so could they.

In the lead up to the great event, she was curious to know what the celebrations were about. Telling her it was Jesus' birthday released a barrage of questions — Who is Jesus? Who is God? What does he look like? Where is he? Where does he live? Where is heaven? If God made everything and everybody, who made God? On and on it went with every answer inviting further questions until Annie's head spun.

Until then, for several reasons, religion had played no part in Helen's life. Firstly, her parents had no way of giving religious instruction to a child they couldn't communicate with. Secondly, even after they were able to talk to her, as Kate was Episcopalian and Arthur Presbyterian — meaning that one church was governed by bishops and the other by ministers and church elders — it could have been confusing for her. After all, she had only recently discovered language and the world in general. And although it was through Annie that she knew those things, with Annie being a Roman Catholic that would have confounded the issue even further.

But with Helen's curiosity now aroused there was no evading it. All the same, everyone wisely agreed she should merely have her questions answered in as simple a fashion as possible with no further explanation. There was time enough for that in the future. For the first time in her life she went to carol concerts where she felt the music coursing through her small body.

On Christmas Eve, before going to bed, again for the first time and filled with eager anticipation she hung up her own stocking. Next morning she was awake early and went from bedroom to bedroom wishing everybody Merry Christmas with her finger alphabet.

Who could have dreamed Helen would ever stand beside the Christmas tree, her face radiant as the candles, her sightless eyes sparkling like baubles and tinsel as she handed out gifts to everybody. She had just learned to tell the time by using a cardboard, mechanical clock so her father's gift to her was a very special watch with Braille numerals.

Until that Christmas morning Helen hadn't been into church since babyhood and her excitement overflowed. First, she wanted to show her watch to a little boy in the pew behind them. Then, just before communion, when everywhere was deadly silent, the smell of wine reached her nostrils and she sniffed so loudly it could be heard all over church. As the wine was passed round, Helen thought it was all for her and the man sitting beside her had to stand up to keep her from taking it from him. Annie and her family were mortified with embarrassment. After the service they tried to get her away as quickly as possible but Helen insisted on shaking hands and kissing everybody and the congregation was enthralled by her.

Ivy Green had not known such merriment and laughter in years. Past Christmasses had seen Helen sitting sullen and bewildered by the odd goings on or misbehaving more badly than usual, especially at the table laden with festive fayre. This year, the Kellers held parties without wondering how soon Helen would start spoiling everything and embarrassed guests would make their swift departures. Quite the contrary, Helen was asked to all the childrens' parties in the neighbourhood.

More than once during those twelve days of Christmas, both men and women were seen to wipe away a tear as they watched the happy face of the little girl celebrating the sort of enjoyable Yuletide the Kellers had forgotten existed.

As the New Year of 1888 came in, Annie began yearning to see Boston again. She'd missed Mr Anagnos and Mrs Hopkins dreadfully and she wanted them to meet Helen. Helen was just as eager to meet them and had written to the children at Perkins telling them:

> Helen and teacher will come to see little blind girls Helen and teacher will go in steam cars to Boston Helen and blind girls will have fun blind girls can talk on fingers helen will see Mr anagnos Mr anagnos will love and kiss Helen.

For some time Michael Anagnos had been trying to talk Annie into writing a paper, a sort of treatise on her work with Helen, but she kept refusing. It was only when Mr Keller, speaking more as a newspaper editor than Helen's father, agreed with Michael that she gave in. After all, he was her employer and it seemed more of a command than a mere suggestion.

Although it meant working during the few hours rest she normally had after her young charge had gone to bed, every evening saw her diligently writing. Her head throbbed, her eyes ached and at times she worried over how she would cope with Helen the next day.

There was so much to tell that the short paper she'd intended writing ended up as a 7,000-word document. Mr Anagnos was so pleased that he had extracts of it published in every newspaper and magazine in the United States. If Helen was known before, she was now a national celebrity. Reporters were at the door day and night and servants had to be posted on watch to keep them at bay.

Early that spring Michael Anagnos was journeying south for a holiday in Florida. This gave the Kellers an opportunity to invite him to Tuscumbia on his way home to meet the child for whose education he was indirectly responsible.

His arrival in March also gave Annie and Helen the opportunity *they'd* been waiting for — to put pressure on Mr Keller to let them go to Boston during the summer. After a lot of thought, he conceded provided Kate also went and the visit was arranged for May.

And what a difference from her first journey there when Aunty Ev accompanied them in case Helen proved too difficult for her parents to handle. For weeks life seemed to be one round of choosing and trying on new dresses and hats, most of which were made by Kate and Aunty Ev.

At last the time came for Annie, Helen and Kate to leave Ivy Green amid hugs, kisses, tears and promises to write home often. The long train journey was a new source of pleasure and knowledge for Helen. The first time she had worn everyone out trying to alternately pacify or entertain her. This time they were exhausted by her never-ending questions.

Before going to Boston, they planned to spend a few days in Washington where Dr Alexander Graham Bell was longing to see the little blind girl again. When Helen had been told it was he who first introduced them to the Perkins Institute she wrote him a letter. And, unknown to anyone, she had enclosed an unflattering photograph of 'Teacher' and herself, depicting them as a grim looking, middle-aged lady and a surly, unsmiling girl.

The elderly Scotsman had been so impressed by Helen's letter he'd had it published in the *Science Weekly* magazine, together with the frightful photograph. However, when they arrived in Washington, he was stunned to see that 'Teacher' was a pretty, twenty-one-year-old girl and, from her expressive features, it was obvious Helen was a lively, fun-loving child. The improvement in her since they'd last met just over a year earlier was beyond belief. On that occasion, she had sat on his lap playing with his pocket-watch while he discussed her future with her parents. This time they held a lengthy, intelligent conversation about wild animals versus domestic ones — and Helen had her own watch.

Kate and Annie were aware Helen's name was known almost worldwide by this time, but they didn't realise exactly how highly she was regarded. Not that is, until, before leaving Washington, they were invited to spend an afternoon at the White House and take tea with President Cleveland. Later they strolled through the gardens with Annie acting as interpreter while Helen and the President *chatted* together like old friends.

It was May 26th when they finally reached Boston where an impatient Helen insisted they go straight to Perkins. Before meeting the students she was taken on a tour of the Institute where she was 'shown' a whole library full of Braille books; embossed globes; atlases with relief maps; Braille typewriters. Everything a blind person could possibly need.

Helen hadn't realized there were more than a hundred children there — sixty girls and seventy boys — and when they crowded round to 'see' her, she was a little alarmed. But when they began feeling her clothes, face and hair and talking excitedly in the finger alphabet she squealed with delight. She'd always found it impossible to imagine people could be blind without being deaf. In her child's mind she had believed that if they could hear then they must somehow be able to see. Yet, because they'd been taught the finger alphabet before proceeding to the more complicated Braille, she was surrounded by hearing children all speaking her language without the need for an interpreter.

It had been organized for her to take part in the school activities without actually being a registered pupil, with Annie sitting beside her in class translating the teacher's words. Some were secretly worried this would hold up the lessons for the hearing children, but they were astonished. Helen received the information no more than a second later than the rest.

She did gymnastics and learned to dive and swim with Annie worried sick for her safety while Helen feared nothing.

One sour note in her stay at Perkins was when she met Laura Bridgeman who greeted Annie with much affection then stooped to kiss Helen on the cheek. Curious as ever, Helen reached up to touch her face whereupon the older woman pushed her away and rebuked Annie for not teaching her pupil well. Then, into a bewildered Helen's hand she hastily spelled, 'You must not be so forward when calling on a lady.'

Instantly Helen recoiled and lowered her hands only to contact some crochet work lying in Laura's lap. Again Laura pushed her away spelling out, 'I'm afraid your hands are not clean.'

Helen was so shocked at this hostile reception her knees gave way and she sat down plop on the floor. Once more her hand was grabbed and she was told, 'You must not sit on the floor when you have on a clean dress. You have many things to learn.'

Annie surveyed the unhappy scene with sadness for

both Laura and Helen. Poor child. She'd heard so much of Laura Bridgeman and had longed to meet her only to be rebuffed at each approach. As for poor Laura, Annie suddenly saw her as a prim, dowdy recluse, aged beyond her years. A shudder ran through her with the knowledge that, under a different approach and tuition, Helen could have ended up like that, an institutionalized guinea pig to science.

Both were so eager to leave their ungracious hostess that, in her haste to escape, Helen committed a further offence by treading on Laura's toes.

With Helen's fame spreading, invitations arrived daily for Annie to give talks about her which she always declined saying all her time and efforts must go on her pupil. Her main consideration was that she didn't want Helen to be treated as a freak. After the painful episode with Laura, she was more determined than ever that her darling be allowed to lead a normal childhood. She was not an exhibit for people to stare at and remark on how well-trained she was as though she were a circus animal.

One weekend they sailed out to Plymouth Rock where, 267 years earlier, the Pilgrim Fathers first touched land after voyaging from England in search of a new life. Having lived inland all her life, Helen was uneasy at the rumbling and tossing of the little steamboat but once she'd grown used to it she loved it.

The next day they went to Bunker Hill, scene of the first battle in the American War of Independence. After they'd climbed to the top of the monument — Helen counting the 231 steps on the way up and again on her descent — she amused Kate and Annie by sympathizing with the soldiers for having to climb so high to fire on the enemy. She laughed herself when they explained the monument had been erected *since* that time to commemorate the battle.

As the term neared its end, Mrs Hopkins asked them all to spend the holidays with her at Brewster, a place Annie had pined for and couldn't wait to *show* Helen.

Before then, though, there was Commencement — or graduation day — when school-leavers traditionally made their speeches. That year, however, there were no graduates and thus no valedictory speech-makers. To overcome this, Michael Anagnos decided the young ones should show how they were being educated, and, with the famous Helen Keller staying at Perkins, she could show how a former Perkins' student had taught her.

On the day, after the official opening speeches and music from a brass band, he introduced the children representing the Institute. First came ten young boys, who answered simple mental arithmetic questions. Then three tables were brought out and behind each one stood a small girl. The first recited a short idyllic poem from a Braille book; the second girl also read a piece from her Braille book, and then it was Helen's turn.

The audience shifted uneasily in their seats and prepared themselves to endure a garbled, faltering rendition. Confidently, Helen began to run the fingers of one hand over her braille book. The fingers of her other hand fluttered like butterfly wings over Annie's palm, so quickly that the audience could barely perceive her rapid movements. In fact, they were so engrossed that they missed most of the story Annie was translating about the nesting habits of some birds. When she'd finished, Helen gaily skipped back to her chair and sat down. For a moment there was deadly silence. Everyone sat spellbound then uproarious applause broke out and as its vibrations reached her she beamed with joy. When a check was made later, it was discovered Helen had 'spoken' at the incredible rate of eighty words per minute.

At last the term ended, the packing was done and Helen, her mother and Annie headed for Mrs Hopkins' home at Brewster on Cape Cod, and for Helen's first experience of the seaside.

As the carriage jolted along the road leading to Mrs Hopkins' house, Helen could detect sand crunching under the wheels and felt the tang of sea air on her face. And as with the communion wine, she raised her nose to sniff in the bracing odour of pure ozone. No sooner had they arrived than she was urging Kate and Annie to take her to the beach. Stopping only to change out of their travelling clothes, they got her swimsuit and towel and took her for her first-ever dip in the mighty ocean. But Helen had no idea of its might.

Immediately she felt the warm sand beneath her feet, before they could stop her, Helen raced forward straight into the foaming surf. Like some fierce beast it picked her up and dashed her this way and that as she screamed and struggled to regain a foothold. Kate and Annie lifted their long skirts and rushed forward, but each time they made a grab at her, she was swept out of reach until one wave lifted her high and deposited her safely into 'Teacher's' arms.

Helen was in the sea a matter of seconds but it seemed like eternity to all three as the terrified little girl was buffeted up and down. Up to that moment, despite her sail out to Plymouth Rock, she had had no notion of sea power. She'd imagined it as an extended version of the inlet at Keller's Landing or the swimming baths, filled with calm, warm water.

Kate and Annie fussed round as she coughed, spluttered and cried, all the while spelling out that she would never go in again. It was a sudden surge of anger that helped her recover quickly and relieve the tension. She leapt to her feet, pointed seawards and, in excess of her usual eighty wpm, demanded to know 'Who put all that salt in there?'

The following day, after some instructions, she was back in the sea. This time they chose a much safer spot and from then on it was all her mother and Annie could do to keep her out.

Everyone she met on that holiday was taken by her intelligence, courage and, above all, her sheer goodness and love of all living creatures. This showed especially on a day when they'd been out riding and were eager to get back for dinner, but when the driver urged the horses on, she wouldn't permit them to be hurried as 'Poor horses will cry'.

They had a wonderful time but before long it was over. Helen and Annie were returning to Perkins for the autumn term and Kate was going home to Tuscumbia.

During that autumn term when one of the older children mentioned that she had begun to learn Latin, Helen asked what it was. Told it was an ancient Roman language now used mostly in the professions, she was fascinated and asked to be taught some of its words. Within minutes she knew *mater, pater, frater, soror, puer, puella, liber, lego, scribo, mensa* — mother, father, brother, sister, boy, girl, book, read, write, table.

Helen was curious about Mr Anagnos' Greek origins and, though she couldn't hear his accent, she sensed he spoke differently from Americans. Now, she went in search of him and asked to be taught some Greek words. Again, within minutes she knew *se agapo, pos eeseh, kala, chaere, kalemera, kale nykta* — I love you, how do you do, well, good-bye, good morning, good night.

At the supper table that night, she tried out her new words and then asked Miss Marrett, the French teacher, if she would teach her French. There and then she learned *Ma cherie, parlez vous Francais? Oui* — My dear, do you speak French? Yes.

Miss Marrett was so impressed that any eight year old, let alone one like Helen Keller, could learn in minutes so many words from three different languages. There and then she promised to teach her French and set aside an hour each afternoon for the lessons.

It was becoming increasingly clear that Helen wasn't

merely bright and intelligent for someone with all her disadvantages her intellect bordered on genius, and had to be nurtured to its full potential.

October 1888 came swiftly. After five months in Boston, it was time to return home to Tuscumbia and Helen was in tears at leaving all her new friends.

A few weeks previously, one of her admirers, William Wade, a wealthy Pittsburgh businessman, had invited her and Annie to stay at his home for a few days on their way back to Tuscumbia. Helen was longing to be reunited with her father, brothers and little sister as well as all the animals. She felt sure they would have forgotten her by that time, but the break in Pittsburg was welcomed all the same.

Mr Wade found Helen more delightful than he had imagined and could not do enough for her. Before she left for home, as a token of his love, he gave her a donkey called Neddy; an animal with a beautiful, mild nature that would be perfect for her to handle on rides around her father's estate.

Helen loved Neddy, but wondered how she could give him orders when she couldn't speak. When Annie translated the question to Mr Wade, one of his grooms overheard her and offered Helen a hefty lump of wood indicating she should prod him with it. Helen indignantly dismounted, felt about on the ground until she found a twig, and turning to Annie, spelled into her hand, 'Tell him this will do nicely'.

6

Education and vocation

It was November when they arrived back at Tuscumbia, and Ivy Green seemed so quiet that they had difficulty in settling down. Helen missed the excitement of Boston so much that she kept asking her father to buy a house there for all the family. But, of course, his life and livelihood was centred in and around Alabama, and it was out of the question.

Shortly after her homecoming another gift arrived from William Wade. This time it was a huge mastiff whose tawny coat earned her the name of Lioness. An accompanying letter said she was as gentle as Neddy but her loyal nature and sheer bulk would protect Helen wherever she went. Helen was overjoyed with the dog and her longing for Boston seemed forgotten.

Annie, too, seemed more content but then, sadly, a few weeks after Christmas, her eyes began troubling her again. This was probably from all the strain she'd put on them during the past eighteen months. Her only hope of saving her sight was to return to Boston for treament — a move which meant leaving Helen, the child she'd come to think of as her own.

After she'd talked to Arthur, Kate and Aunty Ev they all agreed that, in her absence, it would be a good thing if Helen had a companion. Perhaps someone her own age who could share and understand her problems. But where would they find someone who could communicate with her and translate for someone who didn't know the finger alphabet?

Eva Ramsdell, one of the Perkins' students, was a couple of years older than Helen but during her time there they had become quite friendly. Annie wrote to Mr Anagnos asking if he could get her parents to let her come to Alabama to stay with the Kellers. It would be a new experience for Eva and help bridge the time for Helen until Annie returned.

Eva arrived at Ivy Green in May 1889, and a few days later Annie was on her way to Boston. For more than two years she and Helen had never been apart day or night, and it was a heartbreaking departure for them both. The biggest worry for everybody was, would Helen's spirit and the knowledge she'd acquired deteriorate under the grief of losing her beloved 'Teacher'?

Contrary to what they'd expected, however, she grew increasingly self reliant. Maybe to allay her sadness, working alongside Eva, she concentrated on more formal studies setting aside each day a time for geography, artithmetic, etc.

Leisure time was spent romping with Lioness, riding Neddy or playing with Mildred. The two sisters were more loving than ever before and walked hand in hand wherever they went.

It was mid-September when Annie returned and she, more than anyone, noticed a distinct maturity in Helen. She was as energetic as ever, yet more in control of her impulses. And judging by the stage she'd reached in her studies — all through her own efforts — it was apparent she was ready for a higher education.

Now nine years old, Helen was at an age where children who had been educated at home by governesses were sent off to boarding school. Or, alternatively, the governesses were replaced by tutors, each one specializing in their own particular subject.

Under normal circumstances, private tutors were costly,

but as none lived locally any who were engaged would have to either travel there everyday or be accommodated at Ivy Green — all adding to the cost. Also, each tutor would need to be skilled in teaching the deaf and blind, and though Arthur Keller was reasonably well off, he certainly wasn't rich enough to employ such people. No. For Helen to pursue a higher education, it would mean leaving home and going to school.

From her first blossoming out from her lonely existence, her parents had prepared themselves for this. Anyway, it would be good for her, mixing with children her own age. She had proved that during her stay in Boston and she had really enjoyed the weeks spent recently with Eva and Mildred.

Annie knew Helen's strong character and her previous two years education had put her beyond the danger of becoming like poor Laura Bridgeman, so she asked Mr Anagnos if he would accept her as a student for a year at Perkins.

Naturally, when the time came to go there were tears. First, she wept into the soft, warm fur of Bella, Neddy and Lioness, then it was time to say 'Goodbye' to her father, James, Simpson and Mildred. That was the hardest part because her mother intended visiting Boston frequently during the next twelve months.

At Perkins, Helen settled down at once to her studies. Now a registered pupil, she was studying every subject included in a normal school curriculum, along with some designed for the sole benefit of blind children.

Classes started at eight a.m. with arithmetic, followed at nine a.m. by gymnastics. Geography was at ten a.m. and at eleven a.m. they had *Form* — this was one of the classes designed especially for blind children. Zoology was at noon. The afternoon was taken up with an hour's walk, a reading lesson, followed at five p.m. by writing. In addition, Helen persuaded Miss Marrett to continue the French lessons she'd begun the previous year.

It appears an extremely daunting programme but not when compared to the self-imposed one at home when she'd often fallen asleep weaving her fingers into Why? Where? When? How?

Helen still needed Annie in class to interpret the teachers' words, and sometimes, in her eagerness to answer questions, her 'words' were scribbled so quickly not even Annie could understand them and she would be asked to slow down.

With the entire Perkins library available, Helen soon discovered she loved poetry, especially that of the American poet John Greenleaf Whittier to whom she wrote telling him how much she liked his work. This letter initiated a life-long friendship between the two. Dickens was one of her favourite authors and she particularly liked *A Child's History of England*, a rather advanced book for someone of her years as were many of the others she read. Nonetheless, avid reader that she was, with her love for animals, no matter how she tried Helen was never able to read Anna Sewell's *Black Beauty*. Each attempt saw her convulsed in sobs.

When Miss Marrett mentioned one day that she had been to church and the sermon was read by 'the Reverend Phillips Brooks, who has just been made a bishop', Helen wanted to know all about him. That weekend, Annie took her to his church and when the bishop discovered Helen Keller was there he introduced himself to her. Like most people, he loved her from the first moment and she adopted him as her religious mentor. From then on, of all the books she loved, her greatest love was the Bible with some of the passages read so often, the Braille spots were worn away.

With Helen Keller a pupil at Perkins rather than a short-stay guest, people in Boston never stopped requesting her company at parties, meetings and all sorts of events.

Other parents of blind and deaf children took heart from the publicity surrounding her. Until then they'd believed there was no hope. They'd heard of Laura Bridgeman but believed she was an extreme case; something of a miracle. Now their hopes were raised and they enrolled their own children at Perkins.

Michael Anagnos was delighted at the Institute receiving all this recognition, but Annie wasn't and was only happy that Helen wasn't the sort of child to be spoiled by the adulation.

Annie had been losing patience with Michael lately. Almost daily he was giving her advice, instructions, criticism and warnings of steps she mustn't take with Helen. It was as though she was still the little girl he'd taken in from Tewksbury, not a grown woman earning her own living in a responsible job. She tried reasoning that he was getting older and wasn't in the best of health. But sometimes she was really angry, especially when he showed Helen off as though she were his student when it was she, Annie, who had educated her. Furthermore, the unfortunate encounter with Laura Bridgeman had endorsed her faith in herself and in her teaching methods.

Another thing which annoyed Annie was the way some people treated her. They doted on Helen but, unsure of Annie's governess status, they looked upon her as Helen's servant, a sort of 'lady's maid'. They rejected her completely, often pushing her aside, not realizing that without her they couldn't communicate with Helen.

Oddly enough, although Helen was loved internationally not everyone in Boston — particularly those in High Society — approved of her. Some remembered Laura Bridgeman as a child and a young woman and how demure and humble she was. They thought Helen should be like that, following quiet, ladylike pursuits rather than being so boisterous and lively. And, in preference to light, frothy, frilly dresses, she should wear plain, dark clothes and be as inconspicuous as possible instead of being encouraged to think of herself as a *normal* child.

These bitter facts were kept from Helen, a child who loved everyone and everything. It simply did not occur to her that there was unkindness or ugliness in people. Selfishness wasn't in her make-up and if she made unreasonable demands on Annie it was because she didn't know she was being inconsiderate. Nor did she realize that Annie's sight was only marginally better than her own blindness.

Without her being aware of it, everyone remarked on her selflessness. How she always took the smallest portion of everything; never took the last remaining one of anything. Apart from a thirst for knowledge, her greatest motivation in life seemed to come from giving, assisting and praying for others so that when she showed a tendency towards organized charity it surprised no one.

It came about when she learned of four-and-a-half-year-old Tommy Stringer, a little orphan boy, blind and deaf like herself, and living in a poorhouse at Pittsburgh, in Pennsylvania.

Helen was always writing letters, mostly to people she had never met. It was enough to know of their existence for her to sit down and write to them. Always, they replied and this way she had acquired a large circle of friends from all over the globe. There were unknown people and famous ones. Poets, authors, clergymen, the list seemed endless and it was in a letter from one of them, a Reverend Brown, that she learned of the little boy.

'Oh, but he must come to Perkins at once,' she declared.

When Annie told her that wasn't possible because he was poor, Helen didn't understand what she meant and was horrified. Why should the little boy be condemned to live as she had, in a 'No world' as she called it, merely because of money? By then, there were two other both blind and deaf girls at Perkins, and Helen pinpointed them in her argument.

'Well, I'm here. So are Edith Thomas and Elizabeth

Robin and we haven't any money.'

Patiently Annie explained that they were there because their families were able to pay and, with each child needing its own individual teacher, the fees were very high. Tommy, on the other hand, was a penniless orphan with no one to pay for him.

Helen couldn't believe what she was being told. 'Well, tell them to send him here and *I'll* teach him myself,' she said.

Then Annie had to remind her that Pittsburgh was where Mr Wade lived. It was about 500 miles away, and Tommy didn't have the train fare to Boston.

Suddenly she realized how little Helen knew about the necessity for money. Her mind dwelled on much higher things, but she must be taught to be practical. It was unfortunate that she would have to learn under such sad circumstances.

Helen was heartbroken. She couldn't eat or sleep. During lessons her concentration wavered. Joy seemed to have gone from her life and never a day passed without her mentioning 'poor Tommy'.

As though fate were against her, within two weeks she faced more sorrow when a letter from home told her that Lioness had been killed. While being walked one day, she'd slipped her leash and headed off for Tuscumbia, where she wandered onto the town square. People were so alarmed at her size they fled. A policeman, seeing the panic and thinking Lioness was a rabid or violent dog, took out his gun and killed the beautiful mastiff.

Helen was inconsolable, even weeping for the policeman. She was sure that when he discovered how sweet natured Lioness had been he would be as upset as herself that he'd shot her.

When one of her numerous friends heard the awful story he had it published. From all over America and Europe letters of sympathy poured into the Perkins Institute for

Helen, all bearing promises to buy her another dog.

As Annie was reading yet more condolences a brilliant idea came into Helen's mind. If all those people were prepared to spend money on buying a dog, wouldn't they prefer to spend it on a poor little blind and deaf boy?

She sent thank you letters to every corner of the globe, at the same time telling the tragic tale of Tommy Stringer and asking if they would please donate the money to his cause instead. Next, she got all the newspaper editors in Massachusetts to publicize his story and so try to raise funds from their readers.

Feeling better that she was actually doing something for Tommy rather than just wishing she could, she was soon her old self again. It even eased her mourning for Lioness. To everyone it seemed that her only concern now was to see how many and how soon people responded to her request. But they were wrong. At the age of ten, Helen Keller was about to embark upon the second greatest event in her young life.

'I am going to speak.'

As Helen spelled out these words, Annie's blood froze. She'd met several deaf people who had learned to speak and she found their voices most unpleasant. By observing others, they may be able to use their lips and tongue correctly but they never could master the inflexions and sonances of a hearing person. What chance had Helen when she was blind and couldn't even observe facial movements?

For days Annie avoided the subject but noticed how Helen constantly touched her mouth and her neck. She kept moving her lips and making gutteral sounds in her throat and Annie knew her mind was made up. The issue couldn't be avoided forever.

One of the teachers, Mary Lamson, had been holidaying in Europe and was due back at Perkins any day. But when she arrived Annie wished she had been somewhere other than Europe, or at least that she'd had the chance to talk to her before she saw Helen.

As it was Miss Lamson came into the room, went directly to her and knelt beside her saying, 'Helen, I've just come back from Norway and you'll never guess who I met there — a little girl named Ragnhild Kaata, who is blind and deaf like yourself — *but she can speak.*

In that moment, Annie knew there was no hope of dissuading Helen from her determination to speak. The next move was to ask Miss Sarah Fuller, elocutionist and Principal of the Horace Mann School in Boston, if she could train her. This was on March 26th, 1890, and, during the interview, Helen surprised her by talking. Unknown to Annie she had taught herself to say 'mama' and 'papa'. They were far from distinct and sounded more like 'mum mum' and 'pup pup', but it was a start. Miss Fuller was so impressed that she agreed to take her on for a trial period of eleven lessons.

The method was to place the heel of Helen's hand on the speaker's jaw while resting her fingers on their lips. Then, when she was sure of the movements, she put her hand on her own jaw line and lips and imitated what she had felt.

The second lesson was learning to pronounce individual sounds correctly before moving on to syllables; the most difficult being the letters M, P, A, S, T, and I.

By the sixth week, when Miss Fuller asked Annie and Helen to stay for lunch, they both sat listening while Helen talked about her home, her family, her pets and her school lessons. At that stage, though, her enunciation was weak and it was only because they were familiar with her voice that they were able to understand her.

Kate arrived in Boston the following day and it would be the last long, tiring journey she would make for the time being as she was expecting another baby.

Mother and daughter kissed and embraced, then, with much difficulty, Helen said, 'Mama — I — am — not — dumb — now.'

Startled, Kate shot a swift glance at Annie, then back at

77

Helen, before dissolving in a flood of tears for her little girl, who tried so hard and deserved so much.

One month later Helen was speaking well enough to stand on stage and recite a poem during a kindergarten reception at Perkins.

Alas, medical knowledge hadn't yet discovered that before mute people learn to talk they should first — and for a very long time — exercise their vocal chords. They were like the wasted muscles of someone who has never walked. The strenuous lessons were actually harming her voice. She never did learn to speak very clearly — but at least she was no longer dumb.

Tommy Stringer arrived at Perkins on April 6th, 1891. A pale, weak little chap, he could barely walk as no one at the poorhouse had bothered with him except to feed, wash and clothe him. He had a completely blank stare and showed no interest in anything. Helen immediately adopted the role of mother, showing endless patience and perseverance trying to establish some form of communication. Although Tommy was only four it was clear that he wasn't the bright child she had been. It was going to take a lot of time to break through that barrier of silence and endless night.

Shocked at his condition, and prompted by Helen's generosity, the Perkins ladies committee began fund raising for him and others like him. They assisted Helen in organizing a bring-and-buy sale and an afternoon tea at which she raised $2,000.

Impressed by all this activity, the board of governors decreed that, with only a few of them in the country, from then on all poor deaf and blind children would be granted a gratuitous place at the Institute.

Bringing about Tommy Stringer's admittance to Perkins was Helen's first involvement with charity but Annie felt sure it had set a course for her entire future.

At the end of the summer term, happy at what everyone

had achieved for Tommy — as though she'd had no hand in it herself — Helen went home, where a new baby brother was waiting for her.

When she was given the honour of naming him she had no hesitation in calling him Phillip Brooks, after her dear friend, the Bishop.

Sorrow and disillusion

Annie had frequently described autumn — or 'the fall' as Americans call it. Leaves turned from green to red, yellow and orange, Helen had been told, before being shed to lie upon the ground or be whisked away by the north wind. Helen had painted a mental picture of winter, when Jack Frost hung about the fields, trees and shrubs. She'd experienced snow in Boston and although *white* was unknown, as were all colours, she at least knew what snow felt like and that it was cold.

During the summer of 1891, after returning to Alabama, she decided to give Mr Anagnos a special present and began writing a story. At first she called it 'Autumn Leaves' but later changed the title to 'The Frost King'. When it was finished she parcelled it up in a binder she'd made herself and posted it in time for his birthday in October.

Michael Anagnos was so flattered that the story was written especially for him and was so impressed at her literary merit that he showed it to all his teachers. He included it in his end of year report to the Perkins trustees and also had it published in a professional journal called *The Mentor*, from where other editors published it in the national press.

At home in Alabama, Helen knew nothing of this. Within days of 'The Frost King' appearing in the newspapers there was uproar. One reader remembered an author named Margaret Canby writing a book called 'Birdie and his Friends' that included a story called 'The Frost Fairies' which he declared was exactly the same story.

Helen was accused of copying the story and claiming it to be her own and was denounced as a fraud and a plagiarist.

When news of this reached Ivy Green, they knew there would be repercussions, so Helen had to be told. She was devastated and raced upstairs to fling herself on the bed, pummelling the pillows with her fists and sobbing her heart out.

Unable to speak from crying and shock she spelled into her hand over and over again 'No! No! I only tell the truth. The beautiful truth. I love the beautiful truth. Helen doesn't lie.'

Everyone was in a state and didn't know what to do. She couldn't hear her own sobbing nor their soothing voices. She was beyond their reach just as when she was shut away in black silence.

They knew it was only a matter of time before reporters came to interview her, so when the tears and sobs subsided Annie and Helen's parents questioned her gently. But Helen denied every having known of such a story and they didn't doubt her innocence.

Since she'd learned to read, each book presented new words to her, which she asked to be explained, so everyone knew precisely what she had read. They did wonder if she could have heard it at some time before she went deaf and had somehow retained it in her subconscious. With a mind bordering on genius it wasn't impossible. But for a baby of seventeen months who couldn't even remember the few words she'd already learned, it was most unlikely. And anyway, no one else had ever seen or heard of either 'The Frost Fairies' or the book it was in so she couldn't possibly have heard the story, even before she became deaf.

They thought the mystery was solved when Mrs Hopkins wrote saying she remembered her daughter, Florence — whose pink sash Annie wore at her graduation — had owned that book and that she herself had read stories from it to Helen when she first stayed at Brewster. The letter went on to say, however, that Mrs Hopkins had never at any time read Helen that particular story, 'The Frost Fairies', and wasn't even aware there was such a story in the book. Furthermore, Helen could never have read it herself as it wasn't in Braille and, anyway, shortly after she left Brewster the book was lost and had never been found.

Full of sympathy, Mr Anagnos wrote telling Helen not to worry. He had every faith in her and believed somebody was trying to make mischief and the rest were just making a fuss about nothing. The stories were certainly not identical, merely similar — as were most stories of that nature.

Just as when Lioness was killed, Helen's friends the world over wrote giving their support and expressing their unwavering trust in her honesty.

All of this helped a little. Helen, however, had finally discovered the world wasn't filled with loving, kindhearted people.

The following are excerpts from the respective stories which caused all the controversy:

THE FROST KING, by Helen Keller

King Frost lives in a beautiful palace far to the North, in the land of perpetual snow. The palace, which is magnificent beyond description, was built centuries ago, in the reign of King Glacier. At a little distance from the palace we might easily mistake it for a mountain whose peaks were mounting heavenward to receive the last kiss of the departing day . . .

THE FROST FAIRIES, by Margaret T. Canby from 'BIRDIE AND HIS FAIRY FRIENDS'

King Frost, or Jack Frost as he is sometimes called, lives in a cold country far to the north; but every year he takes a journey over the world in a car of golden clouds drawn by a strong and rapid steed called 'North Wind'. Wherever he goes he does many wonderful things; he builds bridges over every stream, clear as glass in appearance but often strong as iron . . .

They are both quite long stories and while it is true there are many similarities they are certainly not identical. What is more, the stories bear far less resemblance than the dozens of folk-tales, fairy tales and nursery stories which all begin with:

Once upon a time in a land far away there lived a beautiful princess . . .
Once upon a time in a far off land there lived a handsome young prince . . .
Once upon a time in a far distant land there lived a wicked old king . . .

The most comforting letter came from the supposedly plagiarized author herself. She praised Helen for her story and assured her that parts of it came from innumerable other stores as they surely must when they were on the same theme. Miss Canby went on to say that some portions of 'The Frost King' were identical to those in a book she was still waiting to have published. It was the sort of coincidence all authors encounter from time to time and no one thought anything of it.

Far from being offended, Miss Canby thought Helen was a 'wonder child'. She hoped she would continue to write her delightful stories and wished her every success for the future. As if that wasn't enough, she wrote a poem dedicated to the little girl and called it 'A Silent Singer'.

Helen was invited back to Perkins the following spring to be once more the star guest at the kindergarten reception. Whilst there, everyone she knew in Boston flocked round to reassure her that she had done nothing wrong and that they had never doubted her integrity.

At the reception she made an impassioned speech for funds in aid of Tommy Stringer and others like him. It became a joke that whenever Helen Keller met people they must keep an eye on their pockets as she was always appealing for money on behalf of one charity or another.

On the way home she and Annie stayed at William Wade's home again, where Helen was given another mastiff, a younger brother of Lioness, called Eumer. At last she was beginning to know happiness again — little realizing the worst was yet to come.

They arrived back in Alabama in the middle of a June heatwave only to find her mother demented. The baby was terribly ill with whooping cough. His nurse had walked out on them and Helen's step-brother, James, was seriously ill with typhoid-fever. This meant Annie had to help Kate nurse them both.

Left much to herself, Helen began brooding again about the cruel accusations made against her, and Ivy Green was a house of misery. Only when a terrific storm cooled the air and filled up the near-empty well with fresh drinking water did she brighten up. And almost at once, James' fever broke and Phillip Brooks' whooping cough eased off.

Unhappily, it was then that a storm of a different kind broke. Just when it seemed that the tasteless episode of 'The Frost King' was forgotten, and despite the fact that Margaret Canby was now a friend of Helen's, some agitators in Boston put forward a fresh theory on the subject. They accepted that Helen Keller hadn't deliberately set out to deceive. The child had been innocently duped into claiming the story was her own without knowing she was doing wrong because they now believed 'someone close to her had put her up to it'.

This time, Michael Anagnos sided with the critics and openly accused Annie of being the offender. What is more, he believed Helen *had* lied either to save both their reputations or because she was afraid of Annie.

Helen couldn't accept that 'darling Mr Anagnos would think such things' of either herself or 'Teacher'. But he had indeed turned against them and totally rejected them.

A court of investigation was set up which developed into a sadistic inquisition with Helen being separated from everyone she knew and trusted while she was questioned by a panel of 'judges'.

'Who put you up to it?' they demanded.

When she answered that no one had, they accused her of lying and repeated the question. Each time she denied it they asked, 'Why do you keep lying?'

Even the interpreter managed to convey malice as he relayed the questions into her hand. It was a terrifying ordeal for anyone let alone a little girl who was blind and deaf. Helen couldn't think straight and didn't understand many of the questions. After two hours interrogation the panel announced that as she persisted in lying there was no point in continuing and they let her go. By then Helen was so distressed she simply wanted to die.

If there was anger when the accusations were first made against her, this latest outrage caused universal uproar. Again copious letters expressing anger at her treatment and avowing trust in her and Annie were sent by friends and total strangers, even from royalty. Poets, musicians, painters and authors invited her to their homes to recover from the ordeal.

The author Mark Twain sent a long letter which began:

Oh, dear me, how unspeakably funny and owlishly idiotic and grotesque was that 'plagiarism' farce.

The letter continued in the same vein, ridiculing the pomposity of overbearing officials whom he referred to as:

. . . a collection of decayed human turnips . . .

85

. . . solemn donkeys breaking a little child's heart with their ignorant rubbish about plagiarism . . .

And as:

A gang of dull and hoary pirates piously setting themselves the task of disciplining and purifying a kitten that they think they've caught filching a chop.

Still, it did nothing to help Helen who had lost faith in everyone and everything. She refused to answer the letters and didn't write one for over a year — not even to relatives — she was so afraid of putting something in them that had already been said by someone else. No matter how her family tried to convince her those rules didn't apply to private letters, Helen was too afraid to take the risk. She really believed that everything she wrote would be investigated.

Her studies were neglected because she was too miserable to be bothered with them. Her voracious appetite left her and she was daily growing thinner causing her unseeing eyes to look enormous in her little pinched, ashen face. All the self-confidence Annie had painstakingly built up in her ebbed away. She wouldn't venture from Ivy Green, preferring the security of her own home around her. And whereas in the past she'd believe everybody was good, now she trusted no one except her immediate family and 'Teacher'.

Some weeks went by and then Joseph Edgar Chamberlin, associate editor of a publication called *Youth's Companion*, wrote asking if she would write an article regarding her thoughts on being blind and deaf and her training with Annie. This promoted a bit of interest in Helen. It would give her the chance to vindicate both herself and 'Teacher'. Furthermore, no one could accuse her of copying another author when it couldn't possibly be anything but an original account.

When the story appeared in the magazine her most bitter opponents reluctantly admitted it was much better written and had more style than 'The Frost King'. Within days of its publication she received sixty-one complimentary letters and they were only the first of hundreds flowing in from all over the world.

Eventually the year drew to a close with everyone making Christmas as jolly as they could to raise her spirits.

But yet another sadness descended upon her when, in the following April, one of her dearest friends, the Bishop Phillips Brooks died. He had given her so much spiritual support during her wretched ordeal that now she felt desolate. However, another dear old friend came to the rescue.

Eighteen-ninety-three was the year of the World Fair in Chicago and Dr Alexander Graham Bell was going to the fair with a party of friends and relatives. He'd been kept informed about Helen's reaction to all the trouble and by way of a tonic he asked Annie to bring her to the fair.

It was the perfect solution. Helen was as popular with the fair's visitors as any of the wonders on show. More than that, she was permitted to *see* all the exhibits in her own unique way, by handling them. There were scale models of Venetian canals and gondolas; of Egyptian pyramids; a Viking ship and Columbus's 'Santa Maria'. There were fabulous treasures from Peru, Egypt and other exotic places. She saw the latest scientific, professional and domestic inventions and electrical appliances. It was a veritable wonderland.

It didn't end there, however. Dr Bell and his party were going on to Niagara and insisted that Helen and Annie went with them. One of the most moving experiences of her childhood was when she sat beside the great falls feeling their might and power surging through her frail body.

No sooner was she home in Alabama than she heard that a renowned garden nursery in Philadelphia had named a pink carnation 'Helen Keller' and was planning to name a rose after her as well. That really cheered her up. She loved flowers. Their sweet perfume and soft, silky petals were some of the few joys in the long years of empty loneliness before 'Teacher' came. With her extrasensory abilities she could distinguish a flower's colour by the thickness of its petals. White were the thinnest, with all other shades varying in weight and density, red being the thickest and heaviest. Even their scents revealed the secrets only a sighted person would be expected to know. Quite often now she amazed people with such remarks as, 'What beautiful white roses'.

Having finally acknowledged that far more people had supported her than had turned against her, all that remained was to rebuild her physical strength.

While spending so much time at home during the past year, Helen had noticed what a lack of culture there was in Tuscumbia. Public libraries were a new concept springing up all over the world, and with her renewed interest in life she determined her home town should have its own.

With her mother's help a committee was set up to fund a public libary that would be open to both the black and white population. This, too, was an innovation. A local philanthropist offered a plot of land for the purpose. Meanwhile, a room was rented where the Helen Keller Public Lending Library came into being with as few as 100 books and as little as $55.

She was keen to resume her studies, too, but as all links with Mr Anagnos were severed it meant working at home.

The histories of Rome, Greece and the USA were devoured. And she made such an intense study of French grammar that, within a year, she was reading the French classics.

Shortly before her fourteenth birthday, William Wade invited her to stay again at this home in Pittsburgh, where his neighbour, Dr John Irons, would tutor her in Latin. Helen and the doctor had never met but when they did, he was completely captivated by both her personality and intellect.

Under his tuition she made such progress that he suggested that, as she could never return to Perkins, she should be enrolled at the Wright Humanson School, on 56th Street, in New York.

Unfortunately, just at that time, Arthur Keller was suffering financial hardship so he couldn't possibly afford to send her. It was even feared he would have to dispense with Annie's services, too. When John Spaulding, yet another Helen Keller enthusiast, heard of this he had no hesitation in funding her future education and retaining Annie's services. After proving to be so gallant and generous, from then on he was always referred to as 'King John'. With his financial backing, in 1894, Helen applied for enrolment at the school.

Although it was in the heart of the city, the school was close to the vast green acreage of Central Park and was in an almost rural setting. Its one drawback was in being specifically for the deaf, where they were taught lip reading and sign language, both of which were totally useless to Helen. Wright Humanson had never admitted a blind student before and weren't sure how to instruct her. The prospect of having 'Teacher' accompany her to classes was daunting to the entire staff, but Annie persuaded the principal to give them a trial.

Though mathematics always gave Helen trouble she was adamant the subject wouldn't defeat her. Otherwise she was good in most subjects, with languages her *métier*. She shone in Latin and French and shortly after starting on German she was reading Schiller's *Wilhelm Tell* in the original.

Helen loved music although she could only absorb it through vibrations or its 'beat' as it penetrated her body and sent the blood coursing through her veins. At Wright

Humanson she had piano lessons, took singing lessons to strengthen her voice and later had a role in a school play.

By tracing the chalk lines, Helen was even able to read the blackboard, and staff and students alike were astounded at her aptitude. They loved her sense of fun and infectious laughter and she eagerly joined in all the usual student pranks; often providing fresh ideas for practical jokes.

In her two-year stay there, she visited the West Point Military Academy and while there went sailing on the Hudson River.

Another time, the teaching staff organized a trip to the Statue of Liberty standing on Bedloes Island in New York harbour.

Every day she was in Central Park walking or horse-riding. When the park was in the grip of winter she tobogganed and bob-sleded. There were visits to dog shows at Madison Square Garden; museums; art galleries and concert halls.

Invitations came daily to have dinner at the homes of the Rockefellers; Alice Beal Parsons, a well-known literary critic and reviewer; Richard Gilder, poet and editor of the prestigious publication *The Century*; Clarence Stedman who, besides being a merchant banker, was also a poet. And she finally met Mark Twain, the man who had tried so hard to help ease her trauma during 'The Frost King' fiasco.

One cloud during that time was when she heard about Michael Anagnos' 1894 report for the Perkins Institute. Edith Thomas was one of the deaf and blind girls Helen had referred to when she was trying to get Tommy Stringer to Perkins. Michael Anagnos dwelled exclusively and eulogized on fourteen-year-old Edith Thomas's outstanding accomplishments as though no one with such afflictions had ever before achieved anything. It was as if he didn't know Helen Keller existed.

Otherwise Helen was extremely happy in New York and the end of each holiday at home saw her eagerly anticipating another term there. Then, in February 1895, shortly after the Christmas holidays, John Spaulding died quite suddenly. In the past year 'King John' had become one of her dearest friends, almost replacing her beloved Bishop Phillip Brooks, and she was overcome with grief.

She was also to be faced with another blow. 'King John' had made no provision for Helen in his will, and his inheritors had absolutely no interest in her welfare. Indeed, far from continuing to provide for her school fees and Annie's services, they asked Arthur Keller to repay $10,000; a proportion of what John Spaulding had spent on her.

On hearing of this outrage, Dr Bell immediately organized a meeting to which he invited Helen's entire coterie of New York friends. Everyone not only subscribed to her immediate needs but they made provision for all future educational expenses and for Annie's salary.

In June 1896, Helen would be sixteen and coming towards the end of her two-year stay at Wright Humanson, so plans were put forward for her to enter the Gilman School for Young Ladies. This was at Cambridge, in another part of New York City, and was a preparatory school for Radcliffe College, an annexe of Harvard University.

If Wright Humanson's drawback was in having only deaf children, the Cambridge academy's was in being a school for hearing and sighted children only. The principal, Arthur Gilman, was most reluctant to take Helen, but once more Annie used her powers of persuasion and convinced him she was up to the challenge.

Not wanting to make any concessions for Helen's handicap, Arthur Gilman set her a daunting entrance exam. Although Cambridge was merely the preparatory for Radcliffe College, Harvard's female annexe, he presented her with an old set of *Harvard* exam papers on English, American, French, German, Roman and Greek history.

At the end of the test, when she handed in the papers, he was so astonished at her knowledge and literary turn of

91

phrase he passed the papers on to the Harvard Examination Board for their archives. There could be no doubt, whatever Helen Keller's physical disadvantages were, she had earned her rightful place at Cambridge.

For once, that summer she and Annie decided against returning to Tuscumbia for part of the summer holidays and went instead to Red Farm, at Wrentham. This was the home of Joseph Edgar Chamberlin, the associate editor of *Youth's Companion*. Like so many before him, he had fallen under Helen's spell and had come to know her so well since publishing her article she now called him Uncle Ed and his wife, Aunt Ida. Red Farm was a beautiful old country house with enormous gardens surrounded by trees. It had a boating lake and swimming-pool, and summer picnics in the grounds were attended by all the literary giants of New York. After staying for three weeks the rest of the holiday was spent with Mrs Hopkins, at Brewster, and in the September, Annie and Helen were preparing to return to New York fully refreshed for the first term at Cambridge.

They were still at Brewster when a cable came saying that Helen's father had died suddenly after a very short and painful illness. She was absolutely distraught. No one believed she could ever be more upset than at the time of 'The Frost King' affair but that was nothing compared to her grief now. Her sobs were heartrending and no matter how anyone reasoned with her, she was convinced she was somehow responsible for his death. She blamed herself for not spending part of the summer holiday with him. She blamed herself for causing all that worry over John Spaulding's will. For a while after the funeral she even refused to go to the Gilman school. Only when her mother promised to bring Mildred and Phillip Brooks up to New York after her father's affairs were settled, would she agree to go.

Trials and triumphs

On October 1st, 1896, just one month after her father's death, Helen entered the Gilman School for Young Ladies, at Cambridge.

Accommodation was in little cottages sited around the campus perimeter; each cottage housing four people. To begin with the other girls had trouble understanding Helen's awkward speech pattern. But on getting to know her better they were able to distinguish what she said. Some even took the trouble to learn the finger alphabet.

Initially she'd been expected to take five years on her course, but after the first weeks, when her progress was assessed, it seemed she could complete it in two.

Annie was pleased at this. She was growing weary of school life. She was never a qualified teacher and already Helen had surpassed her level of education. Her worst moments came whenever she was asked to deputize for an absent teacher and would have to bluff her way through a lesson rather than betray the fact she had virtually no knowledge of the subject.

Hour after hour she wrote notes both on paper and into Helen's hand for her to type up later. And sometimes, while Helen understood perfectly, Annie had no idea what she was translating and simply quoted the class teacher 'parrot fashion'.

Of course, it wasn't possible to relay an entire book in this manner so all the text books Helen needed were being specially transcribed into Braille; a lengthy process in itself, but, as most of the work was being done in London, England, it added to the waiting period and the frustration.

As Helen was continuing to write articles for various publications, evenings and weekends were spent researching from encyclopaedias and other sources for both her school work and her writing. And as none of the reference books were in Braille it meant extra work for Annie.

With James and Simpson now grown men leading independent lives, Christmas could have been lonely for the newly widowed Kate and her little ones. Even had Helen and Annie been there, Ivy Greeen was a house filled with sad memories so Kate wisely brought the children to New York. Annie and Helen adored Mildred, then aged ten, and six-year-old Phillip Brooks and although Helen was still mourning her father's death, she helped make the most of the festivities for their sake. Arthur Gilman was enchanted by the Keller family and entertained them at his home during their stay. When Kate was ready to return home, he asked if Mildred could stay on at Cambridge for the rest of the academic year to study alongside her sister. It was a very generous offer which Kate gladly accepted.

In the second year, when she was seventeen, Helen embarked on an intensive study of physics, geometry, algebra and astronomy. She was also taking Greek. Now, although languages came easy to her, the rest didn't. Apart from when she first discovered numerals and avidly counted everything in sight, she had shown no interest in anything remotely concerned with mathematics and here her troubles began.

For a start, classes were oversized, with teachers having no time to give her individual attention. Normal scientific and geometry apparatus was impossible for an unsighted person to use, so special equipment was needed to be manufactured. This included an embossing tool called 'a Braille writer' and a device for making wire models on a cushion. She also needed an adaptor to enable her to use

94

the Greek alphabet on her typewriter. And, once again, along with the Braille text books they were all late in arriving.

Until they came she had a dreadful time, particularly when wrestling with geometry. There was no way of comprehending the various angles and dimensions. She obviously couldn't see what the teacher was drawing on the board or follow drawings on paper. Not even Annie could help her except to try and describe them. But even then Helen had no way of judging measurements and distances. Similar problems reared up in the related subjects and her work began to suffer.

As well as this, friction was developing between Annie and Arthur Gilman with each demanding complete control over Helen — albeit for her own good.

Annie knew Helen couldn't function without her assistance and constant presence.

Arthur, on the other hand, said she should be encouraged to have more independence. He believed all her ideas came directly from 'Teacher' or the books she'd read rather than from her own mind.

Desperately worried over the way Helen drove herself, Annie was always trying to curb her enthusiasm. She pleaded constantly with her to ease up, but Helen was adamant in her determination. One day while speech training she tried so hard she strained her voice and Annie cried, 'Oh, stop! Please, stop!' That resulted in the pair of them being reduced to tears.

Of course, Annie was constantly struggling with her own adversities; dim sight, sore eyes, headaches and mental fatigue. It was due almost entirely to the work she was doing, but she contrived to keep the fact hidden from Helen.

The climax between herself and Arthur Gilman came one Friday in November when Helen wasn't feeling well. It was only a minor upset but following 'Teacher's' advice she spent that day and the entire weekend in bed.

Believing Helen was really ill, Arthur Gilman and his staff were furious, saying Annie had cruelly driven her beyond her capabilities and endurance. They even implied it was Annie's relentless pursuit of fame that had brought Helen to this, and that she was now on the verge of a breakdown. This was a ludicrous allegation. Both being in the public eye they were frequently asked to give talks to various groups, which Helen didn't mind at all. But it was a source of amusement that after preparing her address, on more than one occasion, at the last minute Annie's courage deserted her, and someone else would have to make the speech for her. So much for her relentless pursuit of fame.

Two weeks later, on December 8th, she was summoned to Arthur Gilman's study, where the accusations were repeated. Annie could scarcely believe what he was saying and flew into a rage, the like of which she hadn't experienced since first entering Perkins from Tewksbury. She threatened to take Helen and Mildred away from Gilman's. They would return to Tuscumbia, where Mrs Keller would be informed of his disgraceful insinuations and behaviour.

Handing her a telegram he said, 'I don't think you will after you've read this.'

It was from Kate Keller in answer to a letter of complaint he'd sent her. It gave him complete authority over Helen and Mildred and permission to take whatever steps he thought necessary.

Speechless with shock, Annie gaped at the paper in her lap as she listened to his next words. She must leave the school immediately without either seeing the two girls or collecting her possessions. They would be dispatched to her as soon as possible. His one concession was to let her pick up her bag and put on her coat.

Half blinded with hot tears, she stumbled towards the study door and left the room.

For a while Annie didn't know what to do or where to go,

then she made her way to some friends living nearby. They were as shocked as she was. Telegrams were sent to Dr Bell, Uncle Ed and Aunt Ida Chamberlin and Kate Keller herself.

Knowing she wouldn't be denied entry in the company of such an influential journalist as himself, Edgar Chamberlin offered to go back to Gilman's with her the next day.

At first, she was barred entrance until it was noted who she was with. When she was eventually allowed to see the girls, they flung themselves in her arms, begging her to take them away.

The night before, Arthur Gilman had tried to persuade them to move into his home, where they could be under his control. They had vehemently refused. Neither had been to bed but had sat up all night, crying. Now, their eyes were swollen, their faces flushed and tear stained.

Uncle Ed insisted that their belongings be packed immediately and then he took Annie, Helen and Mildred back to his home at Wrentham, to await Kate's arrival.

When Kate arrived at Red Farm two days later she was surprised to see how healthy and happy Helen was. From Arthur Gilman's letter she had expected to find her thin, pale and bowed with care.

After she'd been told how he had distorted the truth and heard how shocked and upset Annie and the girls were, she left Wrentham at once for the twenty-five mile drive to New York.

In her confrontation with Arthur Gilman she told him he simply had no idea of the relationship between her daughter and Miss Sullivan. Helen was the product of Annie's infinite patience, time, understanding and determination. She was also the total fulfilment of Annie Sullivan's life. They were inseperable and nothing or no one must ever come between them as each one was equally dependent on the other.

'I even consider Helen to be as much her child as she is mine,' she concluded and stormed from the room leaving him in no doubt. Her daughters would not be returning to Cambridge, ever.

Back at Wrentham everybody was in a quandary. Helen must quickly find some alternative to the Cambridge school if she was to nurse any hope of every entering college. Agnes Irwin, the Dean of Radcliffe, was consulted and made several suggestions and various enquiries on Helen's behalf. Finally, the Dean of Harvard University himself suggested a solution. As the fund for her education was still secure, she should engage a private tutor and he personally recommended one, Merton Keith. So, when Kate went home to Tuscumbia, Mildred went with her but Helen and Annie were left at Wrentham in Uncle Ed's and Aunt Ida's care.

During the next eighteen months up to the time of her entrance exam for Radcliffe College in 1899, Merton Keith would come to Wrentham three days each week. He would coach her in mathematics, geometry, Greek and Latin.

Annie was more than happy to escape the confines of the formal school-room and Helen benefited from the personal attention of one tutor. Annie still interpreted for him but now she felt free to interrupt and ask him to explain anything she didn't understand.

They spent a wonderful springtime at Red Farm. As well as the usual gatherings of erudite people from the world of literature, they were gardening, picnicking, swimming and diving in the pool or canoeing on the lake until quite late at night as Helen needed no light to guide her.

Gradually, as the time for the exams moved nearer, Merton Keith's visits increased to five a week. Eventually June arrived bringing with it Helen's nineteenth birthday on the 27th — and, on the 29th and 30th, her exams.

They were a worry in themselves without the additional, unconventional conditions laid down for Helen; all to deliberately create complications no other student encountered.

As though doubting Annie's integrity it was declared that all test papers must be read to her by a total stranger. But when a *suitable* candidate was found, he didn't know the finger alphabet. Also she would have to sit in a room apart from the other examinees as the clatter of her typewriter might disturb them.

As if those obstacles weren't enough, the algebra and geometry papers were in American Braille. Everyone was aware Helen knew only the English version whose symbols were completely different. A chart of American symbols was hastily produced. Consequently, throughout the whole night before her first day's exams she had to stay up learning them.

By morning she was thoroughly exhausted. Her fingers were cold and rigid with nerves. She shivered, felt dizzy and was sure she'd forgotten everything she'd learned over the past two years. The following night she slept fitfully and perspired profusely. Next morning she felt even worse than on the previous day. At the end of the two days when her final paper was completed, Helen's arms drooped limply at her sides and she barely had the strength to rise from her chair.

Less than a week later, however, Annie shook visibly as she translated the words into Helen's hand from the document that had just arrived in the post.

RADCLIFFE COLLEGE

CERTIFICATE OF ADMISSION

CAMBRIDGE

July 4, 1899

Helen Adams Keller

is admitted to THE FRESHMAN CLASS in Radcliffe College

Agnes Irwin
Dean of Radcliffe College

Miss Keller passed with credit in Advanced Latin

Helen hugged Annie and wept with joy while Annie —
who had purportedly pushed and driven her to achieve this
goal — groaned inwardly. Delighted that her darling had
been successful, it meant she herself faced yet another four
years of classrooms, teachers and toil.

The customary interview with the Dean was arranged and
Helen went full of enthusiasm. She'd hoped to hear what
she would be doing at Radcliffe and what would be expected
of her. But the interview wasn't what she'd anticipated.

'You have shown the world you had the ability to pass
the exams. Now wouldn't it be better to improve your
writing and do something original rather than waste your
time and energy working for a degree?'

Helen was stunned. This very person had done so much
to help her continue her education in order that she could
take the entrance exam. But now? Now that she'd passed,
she was actually trying to dissuade her from attending the
college.

Utterly dejected, she returned to Uncle Ed's home and
made plans for a further year's tuition from Merton
Keith — but reconciled herself to never obtaining that all-
important degree.

The world was always interested in everything that
happened to Helen Keller, with journalists forever seeking
news of her. That she'd passed the rigorous exams was
reported worldwide — and so was the fact that Radcliffe
didn't want her.

People were aghast at this snub, and other universities
wrote offering her places. But Helen's disappointment was
overwhelming. From first being educated she had vowed
that one day she would go to Harvard, one of the great
American universities. She'd meant it as a joke because
Harvard was for men only. Never, in her wildest dreams,
did she imagine coming even close to entering any college,
let alone Radcliffe, the women's annexe of Harvard.

Embarrassed by the universal adverse publicity, Dean

Irwin wrote saying there had been some misunderstanding. She had simply been trying to ensure that a degree was what Helen really wanted. Of course they would welcome her at the college.

Helen was elated and, always willing to be charitable, thought maybe Dean Irwin had after all been acting for her interests when she'd tried to talk her out of going.

Nevertheless, although *they would welcome her*, it was almost another year before she was sent for.

Finally, in September 1900, in her twentieth year, Helen Adams Keller achieved her childhood ambition by taking her well-earned place at Radcliffe College.

Sensing Annie's aversion to school *regime*, instead of living on campus Helen suggested it would be better to pool their money and take private accommodation. Neither of them led costly lifestyles, their one extravagance being, perhaps, clothes. When they reckoned up, there was Helen's small income from published articles, her allowance from Kate, and the portion from the Helen Keller Fund that would otherwise cover her accommodation at the college. With Annie's savings and her salary they could just afford to rent a small house and appoint a housekeeper.

A cosy, lace-curtained, chintzy haven, that little home was to prove a place of refuge in the following two years. This they soon discovered on the first day at college when the welcome Helen had been promised proved non-existent.

Indifference would have been acceptable but from everyone, students and staff alike, there was a distinct chill. It was reminiscent of that shown towards Annie in those last few weeks at the Gilman School, in Cambridge.

Helen's only comfort was in making several friends from the new intake — or, to use college terms 'Freshmen' — who admired her so much they elected her their vice-president.

All others tended to view Annie as a keeper, with a well-trained monkey that strove to emulate human beings.

101

One tutor, Charles Copeland, known as 'Copey', actually suggested as much. He felt Helen's written work would improve if she stopped thinking of herself as a *normal person*. She should concentrate only on that which her physical limitations would permit her to know.

Yet her published newspaper and magazine articles covered her opinions on politics, religion, women's suffrage and marriage. And being well known for always wearing her hair in the latest styles and dressing in beautiful gowns, her views on current fashions were held in great esteem.

Still, fearing she had only a tenuous hold on her position at Radcliffe, from the day of 'Copey's' criticism, she wrote essays concerned only with the disadvantages of being blind and deaf.

She somehow struggled through the first year despite having almost unbearable restrictions placed upon her. Then, in her second year, when a message arrived in class one morning to say that 'someone' wanted to see her in the office, Helen felt sick. One false step would grant the hostile staff an excuse to dismiss her. Had she unwittingly made it? Was she about to be 'sent down' — expelled, she wondered?

With leaden feet she went with Annie to see the 'someone'; the man introduced himself as William Alexander, co-editor of the *Ladies Home Journal*.

Helen and Annie were enraged. Didn't he realize how much they were resented in Radcliffe without them disrupting a Latin lesson, and all for the sake of another interview?

William Alexander smiled and assured them he wasn't there for an interview.

'Well, to write another article then,' Helen said dismissively.

No. It wasn't that either.

'Then what is it?' she demanded irritably. It was to ask if she would write her life story in five monthly episodes for serialization in his magazine.

'My life story! Oh, I couldn't,' she told him.

Then he surprised her by reminding her she was already doing so in her college essays — or 'themes' as he called them.

She asked how he could possibly know that. He smiled again and said it was 'from a private source'.

Helen explained that she still couldn't take on such a task; her studies must come first and they were difficult enough with her handicap.

Naturally, every word William Alexander uttered was being relayed to her via Annie, with Helen answering for herself audibly. His next statement shocked Annie so much that she asked him to repeat it three times before passing it on in case she'd misheard him. But she hadn't and as she wrote it into Helen's hand, she shook more than on the morning of the exam results.

'$3,000!' Helen exclaimed and lost her balance so that she had to be led to a chair.

'$3,000 for a few articles about myself?'

'Well, for the serialization rights only,' Mr Alexander went on. 'Not for the book. That will be a different copyright and will bring in much more than $3,000.'

No one had mentioned a *book*, but he explained that serializing her story would inevitably result in its publication in book form.

The shock made Helen so unsteady on her feet, Annie needed to help her to the desk where the contract waited to be signed. Helen wasted no time in signing for it was a gift she couldn't afford to refuse.

Well, it had seemed like a gift and so little to promise when she was already writing the essays for 'Copey'. But once started, she realized it wasn't simply a matter of producing individual aspects of her life that she felt inspired to relate. She must write all of it from as far back as she could remember.

She hadn't kept copies of her few autobiographical

articles that had been published, nor could she remember where some of them had appeared in order to check their content. And, because much of the material hadn't been used, she'd either lost or destroyed many of the preliminary notes made for her college essays. Notes on all class subjects got mixed up with her 'life story' papers and she got into the most dreadful muddle.

The first article appeared at the end of April 1902, and was a great success, resulting in the *Ladies Home Journal* readers clamouring for more. Already she was writing the second one while simultaneously trying to keep up with her studies, and she was falling back on everything. Each consecutive month saw her writing dangerously close to the deadline and coming under continuous pressure from William Alexander and his partner, Edward Curtis Bok.

There were days when both Helen's and Annie's minds spun. They seemed forever to be wading ankle deep in a sea of paper consisting of discarded notes; some that didn't make sense; typed sheets in need of revision; first, second and third drafts. Annie would be reading through them, checking for spelling mistakes or scrambling around on her knees in search of a lost, precious document. It was absolute havoc and on such a day, Leonore Smith, one of their friends from nearby, came to call.

She took one look at the chaotic scene and thought of her friend, John Albert Macy, Harvard lecturer, writer and assistant editor on *Youth's Companion* with Edgar Chamberlin. A quiet natured young man of twenty-five, he was perhaps of the right age and temperament to aid Helen in her project.

She put the proposition to Helen, who was grateful for any help. All they needed now was for John to agree. He did, adopting the role of honorary secretary.

It was amazing the way he smoothed out the many problems, leaving Helen to concentrate on the actual writing and Annie to assist her with her college studies. That was the work she was really paid to do albeit she considered it her life's vocation to assist Helen in every aspect of her existence.

In the space of a few hours, John had sorted and filed all the papers relating to her manuscript and her college papers. He put them into two separate piles on opposite corners of the room with instructions never to let them stray into 'the other camp'. After reading through some of her confusing notes he saw where and how they could be linked up to form paragraphs, or whole pages. He even advised her on what additional material was necessary to link them. His suggestions opened doors to little, forgotten incidents all of which added interest to her story.

By the end of the afternoon he had restored sanity to the disorder and left Annie and Helen once more in control of their surroundings, themselves — and their patience.

From then on John visited regularly and Annie taught him the finger alphabet in order that he could 'speak' to Helen direct, thus saving a lot of valuable time.

The serials were well acclaimed and after the final one appeared in the August, it was transcribed into Braille for Helen's benefit. Ironically, this was the first time she'd read the story she'd written herself.

When she embarked on the book, John acted for her, negotiating with the publishers for the best possible terms. The book itself took the entire summer holidays to rewrite and to add extra detail than was already in the serialized version. With John editing the book, he invited Annie to write an additional section covering times and incidents which Helen couldn't know about or was unable to recall. Letters they'd both written to almost everyone they knew were traced and reproduced.

At last, in 1903, when Helen was aged twenty-three, her book was finally published and it seemed that John's work was also finished. By then, however, he and the two women had grown so close that the relationship was obviously going to continue.

There weren't many young people in their social group, and at twenty-six John was near to Helen's age. But Annie, who was thirty-seven, had known for a long time that she was in love with him.

Now the book was completed, John revealed that from the very beginning he had been extremely attacted to Annie and asked her to marry him. She couldn't believe it was happening. Everyone she knew, everything she did was either for, because, or through Helen, with little thought for her own interests. Now here was this young man declaring to Annie Joanna Sullivan that he loved her and wanted to marry her.

Sadly, she felt she wasn't free to accept his proposal until such time as Helen obtained her degree.

Helen, now that the book was safely behind her, was devoting all her efforts to her studies. In her four years at Radcliffe she had undertaken no fewer than seventeen courses, each course consisting of three lectures a week for a year.

Now her brilliant memory carried her along. And when others were distracted by the outside world, Helen, in her black silence, could concentrate solely on her one remaining target as she neared the end of her final year.

In 1904, when Helen was twenty-four, her graduation day arrived. Ninety-six graduates — the highest number up until that time — were assembled in the Hall to await their diplomas and, in keeping with the past four years, no one took much notice of her. But when, with Annie's guiding hand, she ascended the steps to the stage to receive her diploma the Hall erupted with rapturous applause.

Although Annie believed Helen deserved to pass out of Radcliffe College *summa* — the topmost — Helen fulfilled a near lifelong ambition by passing out *cum laude* — with praise — to become the proud possessor of a BA degree.

After the lengthy and imposing ceremony, people sought

her out to congratulate her but Helen and Annie had quietly left the building with the treasured document.

The blank pages of her mind were filled. The book was completed. A second volume was about to begin.

9

The second volume

After her graduation, Helen was determined not to rest on her laurels. She had always intended earning her own living.

As they planned to move away from the city and back towards the country, the first consideration was to find somewhere to live. Once more pooling their money, and with the additional income from *The Story of My Life*, they bought an old farmhouse at Wrentham, close to the Chamberlins. It was roomy, yet cosy and, standing in seven acres of woodland and gardens with fruit trees, vines and flowers, it evoked fond memories of Ivy Green.

Before long the house teemed with pet animals and saw a constant stream of visitors, friends and family. Mildred, now twenty, was a school teacher in Alabama and was engaged to be married, but she often went to Wrentham with Kate and her young brother, Phillips Brooks. Their most frequent visitor, however, was John Macy, who surprised them by showing he wasn't only a brilliant academic but the perfect handyman to have around the house. He set to work painting and gardening. He also did joinery and carpentry — making the items of furniture they couldn't afford to buy.

True to his thoughtful nature, he stretched guiding ropes from the house along all the pathways through the woods and gardens. This was to help Helen walk unaided and unaccompanied until she was familiar with her new surroundings.

08

Her first public appearance after leaving Radcliffe was at the St Louis Exposition, in Missouri, one of the central states. One of the events was a conference for deaf and dumb people and Helen was swamped by the admiring crowd. Everybody wanted to shake her hand in congratulation on her degree and for all she'd done for others over the years with her highly publicized charity work. She found the unexpected reception a frightening experience — but it was the first of many similar accolades in the years to come.

Liberated from the classroom at last, Annie felt free to accept John's proposal, but with one condition. She could never leave Helen, whom she regarded as her own child.

John hadn't expected her to. He loved Helen like a sister and was happy for all three to live together as a family. It was an ideal solution and in 1905, on May 3rd, when John was twenty-seven and Annie thirty-eight, they were married.

The ceremony was perfomed at their home on a glorious spring morning with the sun pouring in through open windows to the garlanded living-room. For 'Teacher's' wedding Helen wore a dress of lichen-green that picked up the gold-auburn glints in her chestnut hair.

Annie looked radiant in a gown of deep-blue silk, with her luxuriant black curls piled high on her head, and carrying a posy of pink carnations. She had never felt as grand since her graduation day at Perkins eighteen years earlier.

She had no family of her own present but her adoptive mother, Sophie Hopkins, matron of Perkins, was there along with the entire Keller and Macy families. So, too, were all the friends she'd made in her lifetime — with the exception of one, Michael Anagnos.

After the ceremony there was a reception buffet complete with punch and a beautiful wedding-cake — all made and prepared by Annie herself. A side room spilled over with gifts, some from people none of them knew. Later, as the guests continued to celebrate, the newlyweds slipped away to start for their honeymoon at New Orleans, in the southern state of Louisiana. Kate was staying on at Wrentham with Helen until their return.

Over the months since leaving Radcliffe, Helen had devoted more time and thought to religion and felt closer to God. She was earning money writing but felt somehow the Lord was directing her towards helping the blind. And this made her wonder.

Was it possible she had been chosen all along as a candidate for the work? Was it God who steered her towards Tommy Stringer when she was no more than a child herself? Who but a blind person could fully understand the problems and needs of fellow sufferers? Yet, apart from making public appearances and raising money for charity, she didn't really know how to go about what she now considered to be her vocation.

As though in answer, a few months after Annie's wedding, Helen was appointed to the Massachusetts Commission for the Blind. Now she felt she was doing something constructive.

In that year news reached them of Michael Anagnos' death. Helen and Annie had once known him as a kind and loving man. Neither had ever recovered from the shock of his desertion and betrayal at a time when they most needed his affection and support. That didn't stop the tears from flowing when he died, though.

At first, homelife at Wrentham was extremely happy with Annie supervising household management while John and Helen got on with their writing. He was a real asset to her, always searching for books he thought would interest her. Any he found he would either read to her himself or have them transcribed into Braille. When she began writing another book he did all her research. Then, after months of painstaking work, on the very night she hoped to complete the manuscript, her Braille typewriter broke

110

down. Without thought for his next day's work, John sat up all night typing out the final forty pages on his own machine while she dictated to him.

In 1908, *The World I Live In* was published and was every bit as successful as *The Story of My Life*. This prompted calls for tours to promote the book and to give talks to different bodies concerned with the welfare of the blind.

Of course, that meant spending a lot of time away from Wrentham, which neither Annie nor John wanted, but it was all a part of Helen's work and wherever she went 'Teacher' went too.

Four years of strenuous travelling and work around America finally took its toll of Annie's delicate health. At one stage doctors suspected she had cancer for which she underwent serious abdominal surgery. Afterwards she needed a long convalescence, which, happily, meant spending time at home. But as soon as she was recovered, off they went again. Now she began to heap on weight and no matter how she dieted her size increased. Eventually it was attributed to a glandular disorder, which nothing could change.

Helen and Annie seemed forever on lecture tours, and John was travelling a lot in connection with his own work. Always they were going off in different directions to destinations hundreds, sometimes thousands, of miles apart and eventually the strain began to tell on the marriage. Such prolonged separations made it impossible to maintain a close relationship and their reunions were more like the meetings of strangers than a loving, married couple. John had finally realised that Helen would always come before him in Annie's life. She had tried to warn him before they married but he hadn't really understood the enormity of her commitment.

Helen's third book, *Out Of The Dark*, was published in 1913 and, alas, that year also saw the collapse of Annie and John's marriage. As John departed for a four-month tour of

Europe they agreed to part, and the once happy trio at Wrentham was dissolved.

At forty-six, the years were beginning to tell on Annie's sight and also, as a result of wearing ill-fitting shoes in infancy, she developed a pronounced limp for which she had an operation. Still it was essential that the tours and lectures go on. The trouble was, with her weak constitution and burdensome weight, she was unable to do much other than be at Helen's side.

Kate Keller had always nursed a nagging doubt that she didn't give enough time to her handicapped daughter. Now, with Mildred married to Warren Tyson, and living in Montgomery, Alabama, and Phillips Brooks also married and living in Dallas, Texas, with his wife Ravia, Kate was free of her maternal responsibilities to them. So, in view of Annie's ill health, to assist with travel arrangements and other personal concerns she began travelling with Helen.

Naturally, Annie was grateful for the help at that time, yet she feared for Helen's future. Kate was a good few years older than herself and neither of them was immortal. She felt old and far from well, and she missed John terribly. Helen missed his friendship too, plus the help he'd given her over the years. However she never broached the subject for fear of upsetting 'Teacher'. Ironically, because of her concern for Helen, it was Annie herself who hinted that it might be a good idea to employ a secretary.

Twenty-nine-year-old Polly Thomson had recently emigrated from Scotland to New York with hopes of working as either a companion or governess in some grand and wealthy American home. But after some weeks had gone by, and with her ambitions failing to materialize, she was desperate for work of any kind. She must have been one of the few people in the world who hadn't heard of Helen Keller and hearing of the vacancy, she applied for an interview. Though small in stature she was plump, with hair and eyes the colour of hazelnuts. Annie and Helen were

112

so impressed by her obvious ability and air of gaity that they employed her at once.

Polly, however, was having second thoughts and hoped they would reject her. She'd had no experience of the literary world and was apprehensive of working for someone who was blind and deaf. Nevertheless, she stepped willingly into the fray and her happy nature brought joy and laughter back to a house that had been so mournful since John left. Very soon Helen and Annie found it difficult to remember a time when she wasn't there.

As with Michael Anagnos, Helen sensed Polly's accent and teased her by mimicking it. Maybe it was Celtic insight that made Polly promise 'Someday I'll take you and Teacher to my home in Scotland.'

A short time after Polly joined them, Annie fell ill again with dizzy spells, listlessness, feverishness, sweating and a racking cough. She well remembered her mother and Jimmy, her little brother, having those symptoms so it came as no shock when doctors diagnosed tuberculosis, an incurable, contagious disease at that time, which always had fatal results. To prolong her life by a few months she was ordered to move to the clear pine forest air of Lake Placid, in the north of New York State.

How thankful she was at leaving Helen in Polly's care for this was the day she'd dreaded; leaving her dear, helpless child to the mercies of an often unkind world. Yet Helen wasn't helpless nor was she a child, but an independent, adult woman of means, capable of managing her own life. Helen's sorrow at Annie's departure for Lake Placid and her impending death, came purely from love, not dependency. For years they had relied on each other — both for different reasons. Now they must place their complete trust in little Polly Thomson.

Towards the end of the year, though, the doctors pronounced their diagnosis had been wrong — Annie's illness was due entirely to physical and mental exhaustion, which manifested themselves in identical symptoms to the dreaded disease. Furthermore, they admitted, shame-facedly, her laboratory tests had been mixed up with another patient's, who was tubercular positive. The only treatment Annie had needed was complete rest.

Helen didn't ask but she sensed that it upset Annie to be living in the house where she'd once been so happy with John and where every room bore witness to his handiwork. So when Annie came home from hospital Helen told her she wanted to leave Wrentham. She couldn't help noticing that Annie raised no objection.

Their new house in Forest Hills on Long Island was smaller then their old one but stood in countryside every bit as beautiful.

Meanwhile, war clouds were gathering in Europe and on August 4th, 1914, war was declared between Great Britain and Germany. Stories of appalling fighting in France reached America every day. The number of dead and wounded was horrifying and Helen thought of all those young men plunged into the darkness she'd known all her life. How must they feel being robbed of sight after experiencing all the beauties of God's earth? Never again to see the faces of their loved ones?

In her attempt to alleviate some misery, she caused a stir by instructing her publishers to donate all royalties from the German translated version of her first book, *The Story of My Life*, to blind German soldiers.

Although the USA wasn't at war with Germany, its sympathies lay with Germany's enemies, and Helen was accused of being pro-German. Why hadn't she donated royalties to the French, people asked? In swift response, she pointed out that *her* war was with physical suffering everywhere. Had there been a French translation of her book they, too, would have benefited — but there wasn't one.

All around them, relatives and friends had somehow grown old without either Helen or Annie noticing and the next year saw the unexpected and sudden deaths of many. It seemed they had no sooner accepted the loss of one whom they held dear than another death occurred and they were once more plunged into mourning.

In April 1917, America came into the war and the entire nation was plunged into despair. Helen made it her mission to visit blinded servicemen in hospitals all over the country, bringing hope and cheer. She even danced with them just to prove their lives weren't completely ruined, much less ended.

She was still writing articles, but now they covered every social, moral and political issue imaginable. The more controversial ones weren't always kindly received by her readers, but she refused to yield to criticism.

In November 1918, the terrible war drew to a close and the world seemed to go mad. In an endeavour to shut out memories of the past bloody years, people clamoured to be entertained and amused. It was just at this time when Hollywood, the land of film, fantasy and dreams, burst upon an eager public.

Rather than being pathetic, stumbling and groping —the image often associated with blind and deaf people — Helen was a good-looking, sophisticated, charming and humorous woman. She wore beautifully styled silk dresses and smart, tailored suits, fashionable shoes and chic, jaunty little hats. She seemed to be forever smiling and though she couldn't see the sun, she carried it with her wherever she went, her vibrant personality lighting up any room she entered. From a a little girl of the late 1800s born into a world of horse-drawn carriages and floor-sweeping gowns, she had adjusted perfectly to the twentieth century. So, when she received an invitation to Hollywood she was as excited as a child at meeting famous stars of the silent screen.

The object of her visit was to consider having a film made about her own life called 'Deliverance'. A young star would play the part relating to her childhood but if she appeared in the film to enact her own adult life, it could be a roaring success.

Apart from the enormous fee, always anxious to bring the plight of handicapped people into the public eye, Helen agreed.

All went well for a time with the producer and director amazed at her natural acting ability. But as the filming proceeded, they suggested alterations to the script. Some incidents of her life would need to be changed; truth must be manipulated to add interest. Conflicts in personal relationships must be contrived to add spice. They needed glamour and sensationalism. A romantic attachment must be introduced.

Helen was enraged at the subterfuge and refused to permit it. They argued that as the public didn't know the facts it would make no difference and would only bring in more money at the box-office. But they didn't know Helen.

She insisted the filming be stopped at once and angrily left Holywood. Legal complications followed her decision and eventually, under another company, the film was made. In the final scenes even her mother and Phillips Brooks were given minor roles. On its release, 'Deliverance' turned out to be one of the greatest money earners for the studio, despite Helen insisting they stick rigidly to the facts.

Her next venture into the world of entertainment was as a Vaudeville act in company with 'Teacher'. Family and friends were appalled that she should stoop to light theatricals. But inspired by the film, Helen believed that by appearing on stage she would awaken people not only to the problems of the handicapped but also to their capabilities.

Audiences were enthralled by the story Annie told before Helen appeared. They'd heard of her, read about her, seen photographs and the film but they weren't sure what she would be like in the flesh. Half expecting a timid, shy creature who moved mechanically under 'Teacher's' instruction, when she came on stage they were astonished at her prettiness, poise, stylish coiffure and dress.

Smiling broadly she'd walk boldly towards the footlights, her animated expression almost belying her blindness and the fact that she couldn't hear a sound. First she would demonstrate the finger alphabet and *hearing* through touching 'Teacher's' lips. After that she would stand against the piano accompanying Annie by tapping her foot and hand in perfect rhythm from the vibrations going through her body.

Always the performance ended with 'Question Time', when most of the audience posed sensible questions for Annie to relay while Helen voiced the answers. Invariably there would be at least one insensitive idiot asking such things as 'Do you sleep with your eyes open?'

'I don't know. I've never stayed awake to find out.' Further inane or offensive questions would follow, all receiving acid replies. Someone else would ask the reasonable question, 'Are you happy?' to which she would smilingly answer a simple 'Yes'. Inevitably, the idiot would spout up again with 'How can you be *happy*? You're blind and deaf.'

Helen always silenced them with 'Because I have faith in God.'

These theatrical performances were more popular than she'd anticipated and resulted in requests to go on committees and attend board meetings, all dealing with various physical handicaps or general welfare for the poor.

By 1919, all the travelling was getting too much for Kate and reluctantly, aged sixty-four, she retired from moving about the country with Helen. From reaching home in Alabama, she began writing letters to her, hinting at and preparing her for her demise. But Helen was sure it was merely an attack of depression prompting her to think that way. Kate must have had a presentiment though.

Eighteen months later, just as Helen was about to walk on

117

stage one night, a telegram was handed to Annie. It was from Mildred to say that their mother had died. There was no point in telling Helen and upsetting her at a time like that, she thought, and decided to wait until after the performance. But even though Helen couldn't have heard 'Teacher's' shocked gasp, she sensed something was wrong, and insisted on being told.

Many sorrows over the years had helped Helen to master her emotions, but never had she shown as much courage as on that night. An audience was waiting and must not be let down. Swallowing hard, she choked back the tears and bravely walked on from the wings. The tears were postponed and no one in the theatre that night would have guessed the heartbreak Helen was suffering as she went through her act. Only later could she give in and cry her heart out.

In 1924 she became the instigator of the American Foundation for the Blind, and two years later, with a co-author, Nella Bradley, she began writing another book, *My Religion*. Later, with Nella Bradley's assistance, she wrote *Midstream*, a sequel to *The Story of My Life*. It was completed in 1929, the year *My Religion* was published. By then, Nella had become so fascinated by Annie's life that she started writing a book about her.

Because Annie had always been ashamed of her humble origins, Helen knew nothing of 'Teacher's' early life or her background until she read Nella's manuscript. As for Annie, she was having constant headaches and pain in the back of her eyes. At times it was so severe she wanted to back away; to run away from them. Some months later she finally succumbed to surgery again. This time for the removal of her right eye. Her left eye was hardly better but the doctors fought to save it rather than rob her of sight altogether. Still they knew it was only a matter of time before she became totally blind.

Before then there was more travelling to do, with Helen

campaigning for better understanding, equipment and education to help the handicapped lead as normal lives as possible.

Annie was sixty-four, Helen fifty, and she remembered once reading that 'blind people grow old very young'. Quite suddenly she realized how weary and old beyond her years she was feeling.

All the same, that year saw her making her first journey abroad, which was sheer torment for Annie. With her cumbersome weight the least effort was a trial and the stormy Atlantic crossing to Great Britain made her terribly sea-sick. For two days she lay moaning while Polly tended her. Helen, on the other hand, was deliriously happy as the ship tossed from side to side and the power of the waves surged through her.

There were lectures and theatre appearances all over England, Wales, Ireland and Scotland. Polly was overjoyed at being back in her homeland and reminded Helen of her promise to take her there. Both Helen and Annie loved Britain but Scotland's beauty and grandeur surpassed their expectations. Robert Thomson, Polly's brother, was a minister of the church and they all spent a week at his home, Arcan Ridge, a large, rambling manse — vicarage — in Bothwell, near Edinburgh. There Helen and Annie fell in love with the mountains, lochs, rowan, heather and deer and could have happily stayed there forever. But duty called.

The following year, President Hoover was hosting a conference for worldwide delegates of associations for blind people, and for this Helen made all the arrangements for the reception at the White House.

Nineteen-thirty-two saw Helen, 'Teacher' and Polly in Europe and after a strenuous tour of France, Yugoslavia and England they headed north to their beloved Scotland. As the car drew up outside Arcan Ridge, they all heaved a sigh of happiness at the prospect of a quiet, peaceful holiday before returning to America. But as they entered the house, Robert Thomson asked Annie to sit down in the hall then handed her a telegram which she read and then let fall to the floor; her face was blanched and she was speechless. Her husband, John Macy, who was all those years younger than herself, had died of a stroke at the age of fifty-five, while on a lecture tour of the United States. Annie was quite inconsolable thoughout her stay in Scotland and paid scant attention to the land she'd come to love.

Back in America, before the year was out they attended eighty meetings throughout the USA, which gave Annie little time to reflect upon John's death. The end of that year, 1933, saw the publication of Nella Bradley's book *Annie Sullivan Macy*.

During the 1930s, when the world was in the grip of an economic recession, Helen wrote an emotive article for *Atlantic Monthly* called 'Three Days to See'.

In it, she declared that on the first day she would want to see all those people who had shown her love, kindness and had generally made her life worth living. Day two she would start by watching the break of dawn and then go on to visit museums and art galleries where all the history and treasures of the world were housed; treasures she had only known by touch. Lastly, the third day she would spend looking around her own home in Forest Hills, whose beauty she could only know through others' observations. Then she would tour the city, observing the day-to-day lives of ordinary people who believed they led a humdrum existence.

The article ended with advice to her readers to live each day as though it were the last one in which they could see — for tomorrow they would be struck blind.

Ironically, its poignancy did more to raise people's spirits than all the rhetoric and prayers poured out by politicians and clergy for a brighter future.

10

The closing pages

The *temporary* job Polly had taken in 1914 turned out to be her life's work. Within a short time she'd achieved her ambition and was companion to Helen rather than secretary. Soon afterwards, both Helen and Annie became absolutely dependent on her, and by then Polly was totally devoted to them. In time, they were lovingly known by everyone as 'The Three Musketeers'.

By 1936, Polly was no longer a girl. She was fifty-one, Helen was fifty-six and Annie was in hospital again. This time it was with painful abscesses all over her body. Gradually, though, the complaint cleared up and she was allowed home. However, it wasn't the happy reunion for which Helen had prayed. Thoroughly weak and weary of her burdensome body and her seventy years, Annie asked to be taken straight upstairs to her bed where, eight days later on October 20th, she lapsed into a coma.

Helen, refusing to believe it was the end, sat beside her, kissing and caressing her. But without being told, she knew the very instant 'Teacher' slipped peacefully into the next world. The life force slowly ebbed from her hand — the dear hand that had lovingly guided her from her black, soundless misery and into God's living, beautiful world.

Helen had never known such a sense of isolation; not even in the years before 'Teacher' came. The deaths of her own parents hadn't affected her as much. For forty-nine years Annie had been her second self; sacrificing her life just as though she were her own mother. Now Helen wasn't sure she could go on.

Only when Annie's Roman Catholic beliefs were discussed during the funeral arrangements did she learn the facts about her years at Tewksbury. In that moment she realized, 'Teacher' too had know the living hell of utter hopelessness.

Annie Joanna Sullivan Macy was cremated and her ashes placed in the National Cathedral in Washington.

It was a fortunate coincidence that within days of Annie's funeral Helen was due to embark on another tour, once more to Scotland. The lengthy sea-voyage proved to be the perfect anodyne for grief. People wanted to meet her — and to commiserate over her recent bereavement. Strangely enough, instead of adding to her sorrow, talking about it gave some comfort.

On their arrival in Scotland, before she had time to miss the exhilaration of ship-board life, Polly whisked her off to her brother's manse. Robert was a family man with a house full of animals and children; another good remedy for mourning. By the time her tour was due to start she was filled with renewed energy.

As though the past few years' anxiety over 'Teacher' had sapped Helen physically and emotionally, it appeared now as if the Lord had granted her a blessed release from care. The feeling of age and weariness suddenly left her. The older she got the more vitality she seemed to acquire and with it her activities increased.

At Forest Hills, in 1937, she received a visit from Takao Iwahashi, a tireless worker for blind and deaf people in Japan. He pleaded with her to go to his country and launch an appeal on behalf of the blind. When he informed her that only 5,000 out of 150,000 blind and 100,000 deaf people received any sort of assistance, she arranged to go as soon as possible. It was her first experience of the Orient, and she was slightly nervous, knowing nothing of its people or their customs, but any fears were soon dispelled. She received a rapturous welcome wherever she went and at the end of her visit £200,000 had been raised to aid deaf and blind people. This prompted her to set her sights on other lands, when before she had toured only America and Europe.

It was two years since Annie had died yet when Helen arrived back at Long Island from Japan, perhaps due to her long absence, the loss of dear 'Teacher' overwhelmed her. She remembered her reason for leaving Wrentham and decided it would be better if she now moved away from a house that held too many memories.

The Forest Hills house was quickly sold and Helen and Polly moved further north to a rather grand house in Westport, Connecticut. But if she'd intended escaping the memories at Forest Hills, she hung on to the tangible ones. Everything Annie had owned went with her. She even called her new home Arcan Ridge, after the old Scottish manse Annie loved so much in her latter years.

Nineteen-thirty-nine saw war in Europe again which meant her tours were stopped because of the threat of mines and U-boats in the Atlantic. But for the duration she continued her lecture tours throughout the USA.

Just over two years later, on December 6th, 1941, came the infamous Japanese attack on the American base at Pearl Harbour in Hawaii, plunging the USA once more into war.

Helen couldn't believe these were the same people who had feasted her and listened to her pleas on behalf of the needy; a nation that had showed such compassion. In the following year she repeated what she'd done in the First World War and went to more than 70 American hospitals giving comfort and encouragement to blinded soldiers, sailors and airmen.

One year after the war ended, Helen and Polly returned to Europe. Though she could neither see nor hear, Helen knew she was in the midst of immense devastation. Thousands had died. Some had lived through the horrors of Nazi occupation. Cities had all but vanished; national treasures destroyed.

Under the circumstances she felt useless to help and had the utmost sympathy for everyone — and then a terrible blow befell her. She was in Rome, Italy, when a cable arrived telling her that, due to an overheated furnace in the basement, Arcan Ridge, her new home in Connecticut, had burned down.

All her possessions were gone. The greatest loss wasn't the house, clothes, jewellery or the furniture. It was the loss of precious manuscripts, letters, books, mementoes of her parents, family, 'Teacher', and such friends as dear Dr Bell, 'King John' Spaulding, even Michael Anagnos; everyone living or dead whom she'd ever held dear. What was more, twenty years of work on her near completed book about 'Teacher' had been reduced to ashes.

Then, considering the destruction and tragedy surrounding her in Europe she suddenly felt ashamed of her tears over a material loss, and pulled herself together. She resolved to rebuild Arcan Ridge and begin the book all over again. And although nothing could compensate for or replace her lost treasures — their memories would always live on in her heart.

News of the fire made Polly quite ill and while the doctors were treating her for shock they discovered she had very high blood pressure. At sixty-one, they felt she should ease up on her heavy work schedule. Polly reminded them that Helen was five years older than her and 'getting younger every year'.

In 1948 it was off to Australia, New Zealand and — full of trepidation — back to Japan to as rapturous a welcome as on the previous occasion. But while in Japan, Polly suffered a slight stroke. The tour was cancelled and they returned home immediately. After she'd recovered, it was assumed she would retire but she was as adamant as Helen in the work they were doing. Nineteen-fifty-one saw them in South Africa. In 1952 they visited Egypt, Lebanon, Syria, Jordan and Israel. Everyone knew Polly was under a terrible strain and her flushed countenance, dizzy spells and frequent nervous attacks did nothing to calm their fears. She was completely exhausted. What no one suspected, though, was that Helen, too, was feeling her seventy-two years. She was tired and longed for peace yet felt obliged to go on doing what God had asked of her.

In 1953, another film was made about her life. This time it was a documentary called 'The Unconquered', for which Helen's full co-operation was needed regarding all the facts. When it was finished she set off for South America.

Two years later, when she was a white-haired lady of seventy-five, her twice-written book *Teacher* was completed and published. Months later she went to India and then back to Japan.

She also achieved a childhood ambition. As a woman she was never permitted to enter Harvard University, but in that year they bestowed an honorary degree upon her — the first ever granted to a woman.

They were in Scandinavia in 1957 when Polly collapsed with another stroke and, at seventy-two, she was finally forced into retirement.

'The Miracle Worker', a play by William Gibson in tribute to Annie, appeared on Broadway at this time and was so well received it went on to be made into a film. 'The Miracle Worker' became the best known and best loved of all the books, plays and films about Helen Keller and Annie Sullivan.

Over the Christmas and New Year of 1959 and throughout the following spring, Polly Thomson was in hospital. Helen called to see her daily. Then on March 21st, 1960, as she was dressing in readiness for her visit, word came that Polly had died. She was seventy-five.

After her funeral, Helen sadly reflected on the adage, 'The blind grow old young', yet she had seen the deaths of her darling 'Teacher', her dear, dear friend John Macy and now her beloved little Polly Thomson.

She thanked God that Polly was reunited with 'Teacher' and prayed he would help her endure the short time that remained of her own life now she was alone. There were many friends and helpers to hand — but none could replace the two people she'd loved so very much.

When she was eighty-one Helen was visiting some friends one day when she suffered a stroke and was rushed to hospital, where it seemed she would die. However, she recovered but the stroke had left her forgetful. There was no arguing, the end of her life was approaching and she announced her retirement.

But retirement to Helen Keller meant only that she would no longer be making hectic journeys around the world or indeed around the USA. She continued to work on for blind and deaf people, her home the recipient of a flow of family, friends and workers.

Gradually she grew weaker, was unable to walk unaided and became mentally confused. On June 1st, 1968, three weeks before her eighty-eighth birthday, Helen died.

Helen Keller, the frightened, bewildered little girl who stood on a vine-strewn verandah, holding out her hand appealing for help, was finally led out of her black and soundless prison under the guiding and loving influence of 'Teacher', *The Miracle Worker*.

She wrote fourteen books of her own — and the books written about her are too numerous to mention.

She travelled round the world many times, making extensive lecture tours in the five continents, being entertained by royalty and presidents.

She was on the board of the Massachusetts Commission for the Blind and was founder of the American Foundation for the Blind. Along with many other organizations world-wide, she was involved in England's Royal National

Institute for the Blind; the Royal Commonwealth Society for the Blind, and the Home for Blind Girls, in Bethlehem. Several establishments bear her name. Built in her honour, all over the world can be found such places as Helen Keller House in Jerusalem. But perhaps the most fitting tribute of all was when a new administration building at the Perkins Institute in Boston, Massachusetts, was given the name

THE KELLER-MACY COTTAGE
DEDICATED TO HELEN KELLER AND
ANNIE SULLIVAN MACY